The

7-DAY LOW-CARB
RESCUE AND RECOVERY PLAN

For Every Low-Carb Dieter—On Any Program—
Who Needs Real Help—Right Now

Other Books by Drs. Rachael and Richard Heller

The Carbohydrate Addict's LifeSpan Program

The Carbohydrate Addict's Carbohydrate Counter

The Carbohydrate Addict's Cookbook

The Carbohydrate Addict's Fat Counter

The Carbohydrate Addict's Calorie Counter

The Carbohydrate Addict's Healthy Heart Program

The Carbohydrate Addict's Gram Counter

The Carbohydrate Addict's Healthy for Life Plan

The Carbohydrate Addict's Program for Success

Carbohydrate-Addicted Kids

The

7-DAY LOW-CARB
RESCUE AND RECOVERY PLAN

For Every Low-Carb Dieter—On Any Program—
Who Needs Real Help—Right Now

Rachael F. Heller, M.A., M.Ph., Ph.D.

Assistant Clinical Professor, Mount Sinai School of Medicine, New York, retired;
Assistant Professor, Graduate Center of the City University of New York,
Department of Biomedical Sciences, retired

Richard F. Heller, M.S., Ph.D.

Professor, Mount Sinai School of Medicine, New York, retired;
Professor, Graduate Center of the City University of New York,
Department of Biomedical Sciences, retired;
Professor Emeritus, City University of New York

DUTTON

DUTTON
Published by Penguin Group (USA) Inc.
375 Hudson Street, New York, New York 10014, U.S.A.
Penguin Books Ltd, Registered Offices: 80 Strand, London WC2R 0RL, England
Penguin Books Australia Ltd, 250 Camberwell Road,
Camberwell, Victoria 3124, Australia
Penguin Books Canada Ltd, 10 Alcorn Avenue, Toronto, Ontario, Canada M4V 3B2
Penguin Books (NZ) Ltd, Cnr Rosedale and Airborne Roads,
Albany, Auckland 1310, New Zealand

Published by Dutton, a member of Penguin Group (USA) Inc.

First printing, May 2004
1   3   5   7   9   10   8   6   4   2

🏃 REGISTERED TRADEMARK—MARCA REGISTRADA

Entenmann's is a registered trademark of Entenmann's Inc.

Godiva is a registered trademark of Godiva Chocolatier, Inc.

LIBRARY OF CONGRESS CATALOGING-IN-PUBLICATION DATA
has been applied for.

ISBN: 0-525-94841-4

Printed in the United States of America
Set in Garamond Light
Designed by Eve Kirch

The information in this book reflects the authors' experiences and is not intended to replace medical advice. It is not the intent of the authors to diagnose or prescribe nor to recommend or suggest the appropriateness or safety of low-carb dieting. The intent is only to offer information to help you cooperate with your physician in your mutual quest for desirable health. Only your physician can determine whether or not this plan and/or low-carb dieting are appropriate for you. Before embarking on this or any other plan, or low-carb dieting in general, you should consult your physician. In addition to regular checkups and supervision, any questions or symptoms should be addressed to your physician. In the event you use this information without your physician's approval, you are prescribing for yourself, and the publisher and authors assume no responsibility.

As with any plan, one size cannot fit all, and your plan should be individualized in conjunction with your physician. It is important that together you develop your own specific plan based on his/her advice and your own particular requirements and preferences, so that you may derive the best benefit from this plan.

Do not mix and match guidelines from this plan with recommendations from other plans. Your personal physician should guide you; let your physician help you and make important suggestions. Bring this book to your physician's office. Have your physician read it and understand the plan and advise you. As in all matters, your physician's recommendations should be primary.

This plan is not intended for those with medical problems, for pregnant or nursing women, or for children or teens. Their needs are so specialized that they cannot be addressed here.

The dialogue, quotes, biographical facts, and anecdotes recounted in this book are actual and true to life. They come from hundreds of interviews. No individual has been directly quoted, or described, unless specific written permission was obtained. All names used in this book, other than scientific researchers, have been changed to protect anonymity.

NOTICE: The terms "Reward Meal," "The Carbohydrate Addict's Diet," and derivatives and abbreviations are registered and service trademarks owned by Drs. Richard and Rachael Heller and cannot be used without their written permission.

To all of us who have been told too often
to "just eat sensibly"

Contents

Acknowledgments

We wish to express our deep appreciation to:

Mel Berger, Senior Vice President, William Morris Agency. His thoughtful and incisive advice, exceptional mind, creativity, commitment, and vision make him the best agent in the world. In addition, his amazing insight and brilliant sense of humor never fail to amaze us.

Carole Baron, President of Dutton, whose well-respected experience, thought, and energy have been invaluable.

Sandy Rosen, our good friend and brilliant counselor (in every sense of the word).

Kara Welsh, Publisher, New American Library, and Brian Tart, Editorial Director, Dutton Books, for their unswerving commitment to excellence in publishing and to bringing to low-carb dieters—without delay—the information they need to separate the real from the hype.

Liz Perl, Vice President and Director of Marketing, New American Library, our beloved publicist, who has worked tirelessly and intelligently on so many of our projects, getting vital information to those who needed it when they needed it. She is a joy to know and work with. Her energy, fine professional judgment, and unswerving commitment make her one in a trillion.

Ellen Edwards, Senior Editor, New American Library, our wonderful editor, for her relentless work under pressure, untiring interest, concern, commitment, and willingness to go the extra mile (time and time again) to get the job done (and done with excellence). Beyond all she does every day, for her brilliant editing.

Susan Schwartz, Managing Editor of Dutton, who gets it all together and makes it all work—beautifully.

Anthony Ramondo, Art Director, New American Library, who takes old photos and partial ideas, sprinkles them with imagination, creativity, and pixie dust, and makes magic.

Eric Lupfer, Mel Berger's most capable and intelligent assistant, for his trusted reliability and unflagging involvement.

Craig Burke, Director of Publicity, New American Library, whose excellence and hard work are greatly appreciated.

Heather Connor, Publicist, New American Library, our affable, tireless, and brilliant liaison to the media and the world.

Serena Jones, Editorial Assistant to Ellen Edwards, for her continued attention and tireless help (even while being challenged with a world of other demands).

Liz Perl's wonderful staff of publicists and marketing assistants at New American Library, who are always there when we need them most to do the work they do so well.

The Apple Computer Company and their support staff, for the development, care and "feeding" of our user-friendly Macintosh laptops and desktops that have made our lives a joy. They have been invaluable tools in all of our work. Apple's excellent repair team keeps us up and running, and Apple's patient support staff regularly leads us out of the dark tech forest into the light. Apple's hard work and high standards have made our work both easy and productive. Because of Apple, we're proud to say, we don't do Windows.

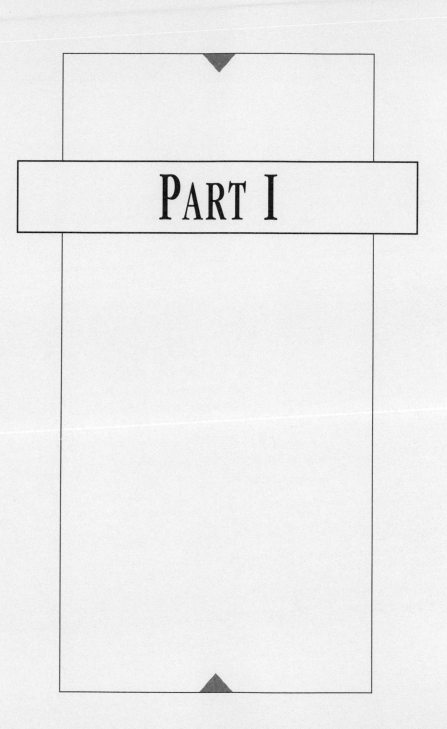

PART I

Chapter 1

STRAIGHT TALK

Looking For Self-Blame? Forget It!
Looking For Help? You've Found It!

Okay, so you blew it. You fell off your low-carb diet and now you can't seem to get back on it. Or you go on and off, never able to get a permanent handle on your eating, or to fully regain your discipline and self-control. You might be struggling to get to that "no-cravings place" you once knew, or keep hearing other low-carb dieters talk about. Or maybe you've stopped losing weight at the gratifying rate you enjoyed when you first went on your diet, and your motivation is slipping away. Perhaps you're starting to wonder if you'll ever achieve your ultimate weight-loss goal.

> Regaining quickly?
> You'll probably lose it quickly!
> Regaining slowly?
> You only need some fine-tuning!

First, some good news. We have discovered that the more quickly you regain weight after going off a diet, the more quickly you can lose it again, once you are back on your program. On the other hand, if you've been watching the pounds return slowly, chances are you need to fine-tune a few elements of your diet to swing the scale back in your favor.

So no matter what your experience on your low-carb diet has been, no matter where you are now in your journey toward ideal weight, we can help you figure out what's happened to derail your low-carb diet and help you get back on track—fast.

Chances are you fell off the low-carb wagon over the holidays, when the parties and the sweets kept coming nonstop. Or when you got fed up with taking care of everybody but yourself and needed a bit of self-administered nurturing. You may have lost it when you went on vacation and needed a break from everything, including rules on what and how much you could eat. Or you might have started reaching for the carbs when, face to face with yet another slab of steak or chicken, you felt you'd go crazy if you couldn't have something more appealing to eat.

The first fateful bite of high-carb food might have come when you simply got sick and tired of being deprived of one lousy piece of cake or a chocolate bar or at least a human-size portion of pasta or real bread—things that other people can eat without concern. You might have come to the conclusion that there was simply no way you could continue this regimen of deprivation for the rest of your life, and decided that it just wasn't worth the effort anymore.

Some of us are like nearsighted
people in a farsighted world.
The prescriptions that help others
don't work for us.

Now you're watching helplessly as the pounds that you worked so hard to lose come creeping (or rushing!) back. Even worse, you may be blaming yourself for failing—yet again— while you endure the spoken or unspoken judgments of your spouse, family, friends, or coworkers.

We know because we lived with all of the well-meaning I-told-you-so's for much of our lives.

"I knew it wouldn't work," they would tell us. "You can never stay on a diet for more than a couple of weeks." Like you, we heard the underlying assumption that we were too weak or uncommitted or both to succeed at a diet. We, too, have been on the receiving end of these easy words that offer plenty of blame but no real help.

"Why can't you just eat sensibly—like I do?" Like you, we wanted to scream that if we could eat sensibly, we wouldn't have a weight problem. Yep, we've been there too. It's a wonder more dieters don't get violent!

The undeniable truth is that for those of us who are particularly sensitive to carbohydrates, conventional dieting wisdom *may simply not apply.* (Some of us are like nearsighted people in a farsighted world. The prescriptions that help others don't work for us.) Actually, traditional advice often seems to make things worse.

So where does that leave you? Well, not between a carb and a hard place like you might assume.

> Most low-carb dieters give up because
> they have nowhere to turn for help.

People fail on low-carb diets *not* because they fall off their program. They fail because they give up, and they usually give up because they simply don't know what else to do.

So if you expect someone else to blame you for failing *yet again*, don't look at us. You haven't failed. You are here, reading these pages, ready to learn about a plan designed to help you succeed in staying on your program and keeping off the weight.

You are like a musician who is learning a new piece of music; you can't possibly be expected to play the work perfectly from the start. It takes time—and practice!—to get it right. So you've picked up this book to learn more about the tips, tricks, secrets, and solutions that have helped us, and so many others, take the weight off and keep it off. We think that's the best thing in the world you could have done for yourself.

Rachael:

After half a lifetime of needless struggle, both of us discovered the physical cause of our inability to control our eating and our weight. I lost over 165 pounds. More importantly, I've kept the weight off for more than two decades.

Today, at size 8 (from a former size 24½), I enjoy all the pleasure of having a healthy, slim, energetic, and active body that I never (ever!) thought possible. Richard, who lost 45 pounds, 4½ inches off his waist, and now looks like a "tall drink of water," enjoys optimal health. He needs no medications and has the blood pressure level, blood fat profile, and all around good health of an eighteen-year-old. When people first meet Richard, they can hardly believe that he ever had a weight problem, although, as he puts it, what once seemed like a hopeless and never-ending struggle is burned into his memory.

Independently, and then together, we have successfully navigated the Low-Carb School of Hard Knocks. It took an amazing amount of learning—the hard way—but we graduated with flying colors. We've kept the weight off without struggle and without deprivation (who could struggle for twenty years?). The techniques and strategies we mastered along the way have not only saved our lives, and helped thousands of others, but also made each day far more worth living.

Richard:

In the first years after each of us lost weight, we couldn't be absolutely certain that the breakthrough approach we had discovered was why we had succeeded in controlling our carbs, taking the weight off, and keeping it off when others had not. We knew that neither of us had a will of iron. After all, Rachael was still the woman who had failed at every diet known to humankind and had weighed over three hundred pounds for twenty years, and I was still the guy who could easily down a large Entenmann's crumb cake and a quart of orange juice as a snack. No, wills of steel could not account for our success.

The only explanation for our health and weight-loss victories had to be our unique approach to low-carb eating. As professors and researchers at New York's Mount Sinai School of Medicine at the time, we began to share our most private secrets and personal techniques of successful low-carb dieting with the hospital's medical staff, our medical students, fellow professors, research subjects, and the readers of our Carbohydrate Addict's weight-loss books. The response was astounding.

> Low-carb dieters, old and new,
> were discovering that they could
> control their eating and their weight—
> sometimes for the first time in their lives.

Rachael:

By using our own personal rescue and recovery strategies, colleagues, patients, research subjects, and readers alike—some of them low-carb dieters who had failed countless times before, and others who had never tried a low-carb diet—were discovering their own ability to control their eating and their weight—often for the first time in their lives.

Vacation challenges, holiday party temptations, friendly saboteurs, the rigors of restaurant eating, stress, time demands, slumps in motivation, and even carb cravings lost their power in the face of the simple tricks and strategies we had developed to help ourselves. Unyielding weight plateaus that felt like impossible impasses were transformed into exciting victories.

Our techniques were effective, and most of all, they did not require the energy and deprivation so many low-carb dieters had come to expect. Letters poured in with stories of struggle-free weight loss. Physicians reported a rapidly growing list of health improvements and weight-loss successes among their patients (and, they added, among themselves and their family members).

Richard:

Some of our discoveries flew in the face of common sense. They contradicted the tried-and-untrue advice that never seemed to change but also never seemed to work. At first, our unorthodox solutions surprised people—even shocked them, and our tips and suggestions amused and intrigued them. In the end, however, our innovative ways of taking control inspired people to think outside the dieting box and to discover that they, too, could conquer the challenges of low-carb dieting once and for all.

> We have walked the same path
> that you walk now,
> struggled with many of the same problems,
> stopped at the same crossroads,
> and today we fly free.

The suggestions, advice, tips, tricks, and secrets you find in this book may surprise you as well. Almost certainly some of them will run counter to the "but I always heard the opposite" statements that may still echo in your head. It is our hope, however, that you take our techniques and strategies for a trial run; try them out with an open mind and heart—with a willingness to put aside (at least for the moment!) the old rules that simply haven't worked for you in the past.

We have walked the same path that you walk now, struggled with many of the same problems, stopped at the same crossroads, and today we fly free. Our wish is that you, too, discover the happiness and freedom we have found.

We want the same for you.

In The Pages That Follow You Will Find:

➤ OUR 7-DAY JUMP-START PLAN

Day by day, we'll tell you how to bring your blood sugar and insulin levels back into balance so that your cravings drop and motivation soars as you get control over your eating and your weight. Each day, you'll make another small change, building on the success of the day before until, almost without trying, you are back in control and right on track.

➤ HEALTHY SELFISHNESS

Your mother-in-law baked a cake and urges you to have "just one little bite." You show up at a friend's house for dinner only to find that the low-carb meal you were promised is laced with high-carb food you can't possibly eat without going off your program. You're faced with starvation or stuffing down the food—and your anger. This chapter provides motivation to help you put yourself and your needs first. For all low-carb dieters who are embarrassed or hesitant to reach for what they need to succeed.

➤ FIVE VITAL CLUES LOW-CARB DIET DOCTORS MISS

In the last few years, exciting research has revealed new discoveries that suggest why some low-carb dieters fail to lose weight. If you've tried to be faithful to your diet, yet success eludes you, this chapter may offer the crucial information you've been missing. The key to your breakthrough may lie here!

➤ HIDDEN CARBS . . . WAITING TO POUNCE

The greatest cause of low-carb slipups, cheats, weight-loss plateaus, and eventual failure is not loss of willpower . . . not a failure of motivation . . . not even interference by friends, family, spouses, or kids. The greatest cause of low-carb crashes are the foods dieters *think* are low-carb but aren't. It's bad enough to eat that éclair (or two) because you want it, knowing that it isn't on your program and that you are willing (at the moment) to take responsibility for the consequences. But how does it feel to know that the vegetable you've been eating might be more damaging to your diet than the éclair could ever possibly be? The ways in which hidden carbs cloak themselves and wait to pounce are sure to astound you!

➤ TAMING THE HUNGER HORMONE

Warning signs that tell you when you're heading for trouble and what to do right away! Rescue and recovery when you need it most.

➤ TROUBLESHOOTING

The tricks, tips, and secrets that now-slim low-carb dieters use to get back on their eating programs and stay there without struggle. How to deal with constipation, willpower hijackers, the breakfast dilemma, spousal sabotage, and more. When you face hard times and harder choices, this chapter is like a friend by your side—every step of the way! We've been there, dealt with that, and here's how we came out on top.

➤ RESTAURANT TACTICS: SURPRISING STRATEGIES THAT REALLY WORK

It doesn't pay to fight 'em but you can still lick 'em! Knowing the way restaurants work (and don't work), and the limitations under which waiters and waitresses operate, can make the difference between a plate of low-carb food graciously placed in front of you versus a grumbling waitress who makes you want to dive into the nearest hot fudge sundae. Time-tested tips that get your server on your side and the correct food on your plate, right away.

➤ RESCUE RECIPES

Good things to eat that will satisfy you immediately and help balance your body's cravings for carbs. Easy to throw together or make in advance, these dishes will tide you over the "I want a carb now" crisis and make you happy to stay on your program.

Chapter 2

HEALTHY SELFISHNESS

We've been where you are now. We know how it feels to fight an endless battle over your eating and weight. We know what you've given up and had to put up with as well. We know how others see you and, more importantly, how you see yourself.

We, too, have experienced cravings so strong that they virtually could not be denied. We've lived in bodies that seemed intent on gaining weight no matter what we did. And we've played every psychological trick in the book—with ourselves and others—in an effort to come to terms with our eating and our weight.

We've blamed ourselves, suffered the shame of failure, and feared that our situation would never change. Like you, time and again, we've paid the high emotional price of trying yet another diet and, almost inevitably, facing yet another failure.

> When I weighed three hundred pounds my
> uncontrolled eating and weight almost drove
> me to suicide; Richard's junk food addiction
> nearly resulted in a fatal heart attack.

In the end, we found the key to our success was remarkably simple: contrary to everything we'd been told, we had to accept that our cravings and our weight problems were *not* our fault; our bodies were different from those who were naturally slim. Once we understood that for most people who struggle with their eating and their weight the problem is a *physical* one, not necessarily an emotional one, a *chemical* imbalance related to high insulin levels rather than a lack of willpower, we were free to tackle the problem in a whole new way, and to leave blame and guilt behind.

As you move through this book and discover the simple oversights, errors, and missed clues that sabotaged your hard work at low-carb dieting, as you see your success grow with each passing day of our 7-Day Jump-Start Plan, it is our hope that you, too, will be able to leave the guilt and self-blame behind. You've been waiting a long time to feel good about yourself and you deserve it.

> We are born knowing exactly what we want.
> Over time, however, our experience changes.

Parallel Roads

Rachael:

When I weighed three hundred pounds, my uncontrolled eating and excessive weight almost drove me to suicide. Richard's junk food addiction nearly resulted in a fatal heart attack. For us, controlling our carbs was not a matter of choice, it was truly a matter of life or death.

If you were sitting in our living room with us, or across the dining room table, we could all share our stories and discover the parallel roads that we have traveled. Since we can't be with you in person, consider us there in spirit through these pages. This chapter, in particular, symbolizes our hands held out in friendship as you take steps toward the wonderful experiences that life has to offer you. In the pages that follow, focus on yourself. Listen to your own story. Understand how hard you have tried and are still trying. Honor that part of yourself. Give it the respect it has earned. Make the commitment to be good to yourself—and to appreciate all that you are.

Know that you deserve the best life has to give. Reach out as far as you possibly can and grab for the gold ring on the carousel. We did it, we got the ring, and it wasn't half as hard as we thought it would be. Now we've come back to share all we've learned with you. We did it, and we know you can too.

Richard:

We are born knowing exactly what we want. When we are hungry or thirsty, hot or cold, wet or tired, we cry and someone comes to feed us, change us, and make everything safe and warm and good again. We learn that our needs are important to someone who loves us.

Eventually, however, there comes a time when we cry and no one comes. We are left to our hunger, thirst, and pain. We experience what it means to be helpless and alone.

As we grow, we learn how and when to ask for what we want in order to best secure what we need. We learn to manipulate the world, and the people around us. And we learn, as well, that if no one is listening to us, it doesn't pay to listen to ourselves.

And so we learn a new and terrible lesson . . .
we learn to ignore our feelings.

More and more, we begin to disregard what we want for ourselves and, instead, act in ways that others prefer.

"Be a good girl and Mommy will buy you that," we're told.

"Just hold on a little longer and Daddy will take you to the bathroom."

We make emotional and behavioral trades. Gone is the hope of finding unconditional love. Here, in this very real world, we learn to get what we need by giving what is expected.

> Gone is the hope of unconditional love; we get
> what we need by giving what is expected.

Soon we get so good at giving that we forget about the getting. In time, we no longer remember why we're giving. Our giving comes to have no meaning except to please other people, and we feel hollow, used, maybe even angry . . . but we don't know how else to act.

That's when we need to come home. Home to ourselves. Home to our needs and hopes and wants. Home to our simple joys and pleasures.

> We put everyone else before ourselves
> and when we can't take it anymore
> . . . we feel guilty.

Rachael:

But we don't take care of ourselves. Instead, we put our jobs, our work, our responsibilities, our families all before our own needs. When we finally explode in anger or when we just can't do any more, we feel guilty. We blame ourselves for being disorganized, for putting things off, and most of all, for not eating right and gaining weight.

Most of us have been badly abused—possibly by other people, but most likely by ourselves. We must learn to be our own nurturing and loving parent, one that fulfills the most basic needs: to give ourselves good food that will satisfy and nourish us, to go to the bathroom when our bodies call for relief, to rest when we're weary, and to give ourselves comfort when the world becomes too demanding or hard.

We must give ourselves the time and care and respect that are our birthright . . . not because we've been good or productive . . .

not because we're pretty or we've lost weight . . . but just because we are human beings and have a right to be loved.

Richard:

So many of us get caught in an impossible double-bind. If we put our eating program first, we feel guilty and selfish; if we don't put ourselves first, we end up gaining weight and feeling ashamed. Whatever we do is wrong and we turn the frustration inward, once again blaming ourselves. Amazingly, the way out of this vicious circle is right in front of us! It leads in one direction—inward.

We have all heard songs and sayings about being your own best friend, that you can't love someone else until you truly love yourself. We may scoff at these statements or find them corny. In the end, they're true.

This program is about putting that self-love into action, about giving yourself the one gift you want more than any other.

Rachael:

For most of my life, I was the girl (and then the woman) who yelled "diet." I threw myself into each new fad with all the energy and commitment I could muster. And although I tried my best, I failed time and time and time again. After a while, no one paid much attention to my claims of being on a diet. I don't think even I paid much attention to myself.

But when I discovered the principles behind this plan, I knew it was different. Without struggle, I was able to let the old habits go—not just the bad eating habits but also the habit of putting myself last.

The irony is that when I was taking care of everyone but me, I didn't see myself as putting my needs last. I would always manage to sneak the food I wanted, and find money to buy the goodies I loved most, so I never realized that what I really wanted—to be normal weight and healthy and to feel proud of my body—were the goals I always put on hold.

If I was on a diet, for instance, and someone brought cake . . . well, I couldn't hurt their feelings, could I? If my boyfriend wanted to keep cookies in the house . . . well, who was I to deny him his sweets? Even if I was too tired to shop for the food I needed to stay on my diet, I could still muster the energy to take care of everyone else.

> I had been so carefully trained
> to take care of others,
> I didn't know *how* to take care of myself.

Sneaking and hoarding food was a way of shutting myself up and shutting myself off. What I wanted most of all was to be normal weight. But doing what was required to make that happen always came last.

People would tell me that I didn't want to lose weight badly enough. It was one of the cruelest things anyone could say to me. I *did* want to lose weight, more than anything, but I had been so carefully trained to take care of others, I didn't know *how* to take care of myself.

> Freedom is *not* an illusion. It's real and it's
> reachable. Don't let anyone try to convince
> you otherwise. We know. We were once right
> where you are now.

Richard:

As you follow the 7-Day Jump-Start Plan, your life will change. As you begin to lose weight, you will also start to lose the unfair burden of guilt borne by virtually every overweight person we have ever met (no matter how much or how little weight they thought they needed to lose). You will begin to lose the pain of past failures and the fear that things will never change. Most of all, we hope you will lose the belief that no one understands, or that there is no way out.

Be assured that you are not alone. We are with you. Each day's Guidelines, every word, has been written to help you, to show you how to be free.

Freedom is *not* an illusion. It's real and it's reachable. Don't let anyone try to convince you otherwise. Especially yourself. We know. We were once right where you are now.

Follow the Guidelines of the 7-Day Jump-Start Plan. They will help to set you free. Write down your feelings. Listen to yourself. Buy the food *you* like. Take the time you need to prepare it. Take the money that you would spend on others and take yourself out to dinner or buy yourself a gift. Learn to say no when your needs are not being met. Help yourself. Don't make promises that will take time away from you.

Put yourself first. In the end, you are the only one you can ever count on to make this change that you want so much. You are important. Never stop caring and never, never let go of your dreams. They are your only path to freedom. When you take care of your own needs and wants, you are feeding your soul. If others protest that you are not taking care of them, perhaps they will learn to take better care of themselves. If they say that suddenly you have become self-centered or selfish, remember that it is the only path by which you will realize your dream of becoming slim and healthy.

In the pages that follow, we invite you to come home to yourself, to a place where you come first. It's a warm and wonderful place, and as we think you already know, it's been waiting for you for a very long time.

In the end, a little healthy selfishness can be a very good thing.

Chapter 3

THE 7-DAY JUMP-START PLAN

First, We Fix The *Cause* Of The Problem

This program has been designed for you, the low-carb dieter, to cut your physical need for carbohydrates by helping to balance your insulin and blood sugar levels. When blood sugar and insulin levels are in balance, cravings for carbohydrates drop dramatically and, in many cases, are eliminated altogether, making it easier to stick to a low-carbohydrate diet without struggle, and to lose weight with fewer stalls and plateaus.*

The 7-Day Low-Carb Rescue and Recovery Plan is divided into two sections: (1) The 7-Day Jump-Start Plan, an eating program that goes to work on Day #1 to begin to balance your blood sugar and insulin levels, cut your cravings, and move your body out of a fat-storing mode into a fat-burning mode, and (2) a collection of chapters that contain essential tips, tactics, strategies, and information that will help you get on track and stay on track without giving up the foods you love.

---

*This plan works well for those on low-carb diets or for those on controlled-carbohydrate diets. For ease of communication, when the term "low-carbohydrate diet" is used, it is meant to include low-carb diets and controlled-carbohydrate diets, as well. As with all weight-loss programs, the appropriateness of eating choices and changes should be approved and monitored by your physician.

The 7-Day Jump Start Plan

In the eating plan that follows, each of the seven steps enhances the step that has come before. With each day, as the physical *cause* of your carbohydrate cravings is reduced, then eliminated, you will gain greater control over your eating and your weight. At the end of this one-week plan, you will be far better able to choose the foods *you* want to eat, enjoy them when *you* want to, and lose weight at a rate that keeps you motivated and moving toward your goal, while feeling rewarded and satisfied all along the way.

> Chances are, you have been told that
> you don't have enough willpower.
> Nothing could be further from the truth.

Chances are, sometime in the past you were told that you don't have enough willpower to succeed at your diet, even though when it comes to food, there have been times that you have shown near-heroic restraint. You may have been told that you don't really want to be slim, or that you have self-destructive tendencies (although you may have tried virtually anything you could to become healthy and slim). Friends, family, physicians, spouses, even your own children may watch every morsel you put into your mouth and chastise you for being weak or self–indulgent. Nothing could be further from the truth.

Those of us who work tirelessly to take off weight by controlling our eating (especially those who have tried to follow low-carb diets), have been told to eat less, try harder, and exhibit far greater self-control than those people who happen to be naturally slim. There's nothing more maddening than thin people who make no secret of their ability to eat anything they like and still maintain a perfect weight.

"Oh, I could never be on a diet like that," they say. "I don't have the willpower."

"Don't push it," we're tempted to answer, though we usually restrain ourselves.

> Intense, recurring carbohydrate cravings and easy weight gain are *not* a matter of willpower. They are simply a matter of biology.
>
> Your particular biology!

Directly or indirectly, most weight-loss programs blame the victim. We believe you have the right to get the help and support you need rather than the easy blame and criticism of those who should know better. Study after study has shown that those who struggle with their eating and weight have a different genetic profile than other people. Researchers have mapped the gene and it lies near the gene for alcoholism and cocaine addiction (interesting!).

The obesity gene plays a strong role in the way our bodies respond to carbohydrate-rich foods, by increasing insulin production and insulin resistance, which in turn has a big impact on blood sugar levels and, of course, cravings and weight gain. The impact of the obesity gene on our bodies may be obvious from childhood or may be triggered by puberty, pregnancy, stress, the effects of medication, a diet high in carbohydrates or Carbohydrate Act-Alikes,* or the simple act of aging.

In any case, intense and recurring carbohydrate cravings and easy weight gain are *not* a matter of willpower. They are simply a matter of biology. Your biology! We know what causes them and we know how to correct them.

In the chapters that follow, you will discover the powerful strategies, secrets, tricks, and tips that can help you to correct the cause of your cravings and to stay on your low-carb diet without struggle. You'll learn how to maximize both your weight

---

*You'll find more information on Carbohydrate Act-Alikes in Chapter 12, "Five Vital Clues Low-Carb Diet Doctors Miss."

loss and your pleasure. We'll help you get past the barriers and over the pitfalls that might have blocked you when you thought you had to do it alone. We'll be there with you, helping to anticipate the diet challenges that you may encounter, cut them off at the pass, and slash them down to size.

> On this plan,
> you will never be asked to give up
> any food that you enjoy—
> so you won't feel deprived.

But first, let's correct the *cause* of your cravings for carbohydrates so that your body and mind can join forces to help you get the body and the health and the life that you want.

Because the 7-Day Jump-Start Plan is aimed at correcting the physical cause of your eating and weight problems, you will *never* be asked to give up the foods that you enjoy—so you need never feel deprived. Each day's Guideline will ask you to *add* certain kinds of food, *balance* different kinds of food, or *delay* eating certain food. You will still be able to eat your favorite food every day.

Before starting each day, make sure that you have read through the Guideline for that day. If possible, it is best to get an understanding of a Guideline the day before so that if you are asked to add a certain food or to make a choice among several foods, you have what you need on hand.

Add On, Balance, Or Hold On: That's It!

Each of the Guidelines is simple and short; each asks you to either add on, balance, or hold on, simple no-stress changes that have been shown to help balance blood sugar levels and insulin levels and/or reduce your insulin resistance, all of which translate into fewer cravings and better weight loss. The purpose of each day's Guideline will be explained so that you can better understand why your cravings are vanishing and your self-control has returned.

If, for any reason, you aren't able to satisfy a day's Guideline, don't worry. Stay with that Guideline and try again the next day. Don't move on to the next Guideline until you feel comfortable and in control of the current Guideline. Remember, this is not a race. No one is scoring you on speed, and the world is not going to come to an end if it takes you an extra day (or several days) to get back on track. Take your time and do it right. (You've probably been rushing to lose weight for a long time.) Reread the Guideline very carefully (it's probably much easier than you thought) and read over the Trouble Tamer for each day and the "TroubleShooting" chapter as well.

> This plan is about learning,
> not about perfection.

Each of us learns far more by *not* doing something perfectly from the start than we do from being perfect. So don't be hard on yourself! (That's part of the old blame cycle that you don't need anymore.) If you don't do it right the first time, pick yourself up, dust yourself off, figure out what went wrong, get the help you need from this book, and try it again!

Remember, this plan is about learning, not about perfection. If you get closer to your goal each time you try, you will eventually achieve it.

Like No Other Guidelines In The World

In the seven Guidelines that follow, you'll be asked to add food to your meals, to save certain foods until certain meals, or to make choices based on what you "prefer" within certain categories. You may be familiar with a more limited and stringent set of dieting rules, usually accompanied by long lists of foods "never to be eaten" or "eaten only in tiny quantities." Such old-fashioned dieting guidelines are based on the "less is better" school of thinking. The crafters of these approaches may not have tested their rules and regulations to determine if a greater flexibility might result in the same desired weight loss.

> Richard and I are living proof that you *don't* have to eliminate carbohydrate-rich foods in order to cut cravings and lose weight.

In previous books, particularly in our *Carbohydrate Addict's LifeSpan Program*, we revealed that the opposite is true: that you don't have to eliminate carbohydrate-rich foods in order to reap the benefits of reduced cravings and easy weight loss. With two hundred pounds gone from our bodies for over twenty years, we're living proof that you can still have your cake and your weight loss, too.

If your goal is to return to your old low-carb diet, after Day #7 you'll be ready to do so. The seven Guidelines can help ensure your success in getting back on your program and staying on it. These Guidelines will also give you a backup plan in case you hit unexpected setbacks.

If, on the other hand, when you have completed Day #7 of the Plan, you don't want to give up the easy, craving-free control of your eating and weight that you have discovered, and you want to continue to enjoy the foods you love every day, you will be able to do that too!

Starting Points

Every person reading this page will begin this plan at a different starting point. Some may be eating high-carb foods throughout the day, at every meal and snack. Others may be sticking to their low-carb eating plan at *most* meals and snacks, with a daily meal or snack that contains high-carb foods. Others may be eating low-carb pretty consistently for all meals and snacks but find themselves slipping or "cheating," eating high-carb foods now and then.

Each of the Guidelines addresses all of these situations. For those who are eating high-carbs throughout the day, the Guidelines will help you to quickly add foods to help balance your blood sugar and insulin levels, break the craving cycle, and jump-start you back into control. For those who have only occasional lapses into high-carb eating, each of the Guidelines will help you achieve the consistency that is essential in keeping cravings down and avoiding weight-loss plateaus.

The sample menus that follow for each of the seven Guidelines assume that as you begin this plan, you are eating high-carb foods throughout the day. In that case, the menus will give you clear examples on how to progress through each of the seven Guidelines.

On the other hand, if you are *not* eating high-carb foods at all meals but, rather, having high-carb foods only sporadically, slipping on and off a low-carb plan, we will offer special assistance on how to adapt each of the menus to your needs. In the chapters that follow we start with your current eating pattern and move toward lower-carb eating in keeping with each successive Guideline.

We think you're going to be pleased to see how easy it is to begin and how good you'll feel along the way.

Chapter 4

DAY #1:
CUTTING CRAVINGS

GUIDELINE: ADD ON LOW-CARB PROTEIN TO
EVERY MEAL AND SNACK.

The Guidelines for Day #1 and Day #2 go to work immediately to help counteract the cravings and weight gain that high-carb foods set in motion. Low-carb protein, especially low-carb protein that is low in fat, can help stabilize your blood sugar levels, keeping them steady, with fewer peaks and valleys. Blood sugar highs and lows can stimulate cravings for more carbs. To offset some of the blood sugar swings that can result from past over-carbing, it's important to add the power of low-carb protein.

In this first step, choose from any of the low-carb proteins on the 7-Day Jump-Start Plan Low-Carb Protein List on page 36 and add at least one low-carb protein to each meal and snack you eat today.

In general, you will continue to eat as you have been eating—including any carbohydrates you'd normally have. The only difference is that today you will add low-carb protein to each of your meals and snacks.

If your eating has been changeable, going on and off your low-carb diet, choose a comfortable way of eating that will not cause any great strain and that is clearly not against your physician's recommendations. Your starting point isn't as important as focusing on today's Guideline.

Don't try to get back onto your old
low-carb diet now. Eat as you have been
eating, just add low-carb protein to
each of your meals and snacks.

Whenever you can, choose low-carb proteins that are lower in saturated fat. The higher the saturated fat content of a low-carb protein, the more likely it is to set off an insulin imbalance that can lead to cravings and plateaus (or to weight gain!) as well as to health concerns. You'll find more on saturated fats and their impact on insulin, cravings, and plateaus in Chapter 12, "Five Vital Clues Low-Carb Diet Doctors Miss."

The amount of low-carb protein that you add to your meals and snacks is not as important as being consistent—add it to *every* meal and snack as required by that day's Guideline.

If you can and are willing to do so, the addition of a full "average" portion of low-carb protein to every meal or snack is ideal. Adding two different low-carb proteins to the same meal is a great way of keeping your food interesting.

Let's see how this Guideline plays out in real life. Let's say that you are about to have a bagel with cream cheese for breakfast. Even though the cream cheese provides a minimal amount of low-carb protein, Day #1's Guideline asks you to add additional low-carb protein. Adding some scrambled eggs or egg whites will make a more balanced meal, in terms of blood sugar and insulin. Add some low-fat cheese as well and you've taken the first step toward reducing those "it's an hour to lunch and I'm starving" cravings.

The chart that follows will provide you with some practical ways of adding low-carb protein to a typical daily menu. Please don't follow this menu per se. It is only meant to illustrate how one day's menu can change over each of the seven days to come.

DAY #1 EXAMPLES

Old *Breakfast*	*New* *Day #1 Breakfast*
BAGEL WITH CREAM CHEESE COFFEE WITH MILK	BAGEL WITH CREAM CHEESE COFFEE WITH MILK *ADD* 1–2 SCRAMBLED EGGS* OR SLICED TURKEY BREAST OR POACHED SALMON
Old *Lunch*	*New* *Day #1 Lunch*
CHICKEN NOODLE SOUP ROLL AND BUTTER COKE LARGE CHOCOLATE CHIP COOKIE	CHICKEN NOODLE SOUP ROLL AND BUTTER COKE LARGE CHOCOLATE CHIP COOKIE *ADD* SCOOP OF TUNA SALAD OR ¼ ROTISSERIE CHICKEN
Old *Dinner*	*New* *Day #1 Dinner*
GARLIC BREAD SPAGHETTI WITH SAUCE 1–2 MEATBALLS GLASS OF WINE PLATE OF FRESH FRUIT	GARLIC BREAD SPAGHETTI WITH SAUCE 1–2 MEATBALLS GLASS OF WINE PLATE OF FRESH FRUIT *ADD* SHRIMP DIJON APPETIZER (See Recipe Chapter) AND 1–2 ADDITIONAL MEATBALLS (for a total of 3–4)

(chart continues)

*Or the equivalent in egg whites or a cheese omelet, preferably low-fat.

Old *Late-Night Snack*	*New Day #1* *Late-Night Snack*
POTATO CHIPS CHOCOLATE BAR	POTATO CHIPS CHOCOLATE BAR *ADD* 3–4 BUFFALO CHICKEN DRUMETTES

On Day #1, you may find you're eating more food than you're used to. Remember that the quantity of the low-carb protein you add is up to you. Ideally, you will add an "average" portion, similar to that which you would get in a restaurant, but if you prefer, you can add less. If you are enjoying the protein and *naturally* want to reduce your carbohydrate intake for that meal or snack—*not* because you have to, but because you *want* to—feel free to leave a bit of your carbohydrate-rich food on the plate.

By late into Day #1, you may already be witnessing the power that low-carb protein has to help bring your blood sugar levels back into balance and to cut your cravings. In any case, no matter how much you've carbo-loaded your meals and snacks, add *some* low-carb protein to your plate every time you eat.

> Each excess pound can be
> the physical result of putting
> the needs of others before your own.

What if you skip a meal? Don't skip meals simply because you don't have time. Making time to take care of yourself is an essential part of any successful weight-loss program and any healthy way of life. Of all the reasons why people fail to stick to their diets, the fact that they don't take the time to take care of themselves has to rank among the top. In many cases, each excess pound can be the physical result of putting the needs of your friends, family, or job before your own. If putting other people's needs before your own sounds all too familiar, read Chapter 2, "Healthy Selfishness." In fact, you may want to reread it before you start to slip into old habits of being the good and dependable nurturer to everyone but yourself.

> The "I have to lose twenty pounds by my brother's wedding" mentality has led to more weight gain than Godiva chocolates.

Don't skip meals because you are trying to lose weight more quickly. Quick weight loss and the quick regaining of all lost weight (and more) are the hallmarks of the professional dieter. We all know the pattern of deprivation, frustration, and capitulation. The very reason for the success of the 7-Day Jump-Start Plan is that it does not deprive you of the food you love but, rather, works to correct the cause of your cravings and easy weight gain. Do not sabotage the wonderful benefits of this plan by adding your own time demands. It is counterproductive.

The "I have to lose twenty pounds by my brother's wedding" mentality has led to more weight gain than Godiva chocolates. The physical and emotional exhaustion of forced starvation can have devastating long-term effects on your body's metabolism and your state of mind. Pushed too hard, you will almost certainly rebound, and when you do, the pendulum will swing toward diet failure and inevitable weight gain.

So put down the calculator and concentrate on following each day's Guideline. That's your job. Your body will do its part in its own good time, and without you pushing it, it will do it more efficiently and with longer lasting results.

If, on the other hand, you tend to skip a meal here or there because you simply aren't hungry, that's fine. We don't see anything wrong with that. One of the benefits of this plan is that your cravings can literally plummet. We have never found any scientific research that says humans must eat three times a day. If you are not hungry, and skipping a meal doesn't result in crazed rebounds of food consumption, and, of course, assuming your physician does not object, we cannot see the harm in listening to your body (as naturally slim people do) and skipping a meal (or two).

Richard and I don't eat when we're not hungry. Because we rarely, if ever, crave food, we eat fewer meals than most people. It's liberating to be freed from a regimen of meals. We're glad to no longer be slaves to the powerful urges that once ruled our lives. If you skip a meal because you simply aren't hungry, don't be concerned with the Guidelines that would otherwise apply to that meal. So just because a Guideline says to have low-carb protein, don't have it when otherwise you would not eat.

What should you do if you are already eating a good portion of low-carb protein at a meal and the Guideline says to add more? Unless your physician recommends otherwise, add a second portion. A second low-carb protein can help to further decrease your need for the carbohydrates you've included in this meal and help you get ready to move toward an easy and more productive weight loss.

> Facing a huge piece of animal flesh on your plate will never hold your interest for long or sustain your need for pleasure. To stay on any diet, the food has to be fun!

One of the most common mistakes that low-carb dieters make is getting in the habit of including only one type of low-carb protein in any meal or snack. If you want to stick with your diet, you have to make it fun! Facing a huge piece of animal flesh on your plate will never hold your interest or sustain your need for pleasure. And you can't rob yourself of pleasure for very long before you'll start to rebel. Eating the same food day in and day out, food that is prepared just to fill the requirements of a diet, is just plain boring. And unnecessarily so. Replace that same old low-carb protein with a veritable cornucopia of low-carb treats and you'll find you are far less tempted to go off this plan.

For some exciting treats that are ready and waiting when you need them, we've included a slew of suggestions in the "Rescue Recipes" chapter of this book. From Low-Carb Lasagna to Shrimp Dijon, from Taiwanese Sesame Pork with Garlic Cream Sauce to Italian Flatbread Topped with Pesto Sauce, you can transform diet drudgery into an exciting adventure. Rescue Recipes offer a starting place to stir your imagination and interest and, with each taste, remind you that low-carb eating need never be monotonous.

For even more recipes to keep you motivated and satisfied, choose from among the 250 recipes in our *Carbohydrate Addict's Cookbook*. It's helped hundreds of thousands of low-carb dieters discover that their food can be fun again.

So grab some low-carb protein as listed on page 36, add it to every meal and snack, and you'll begin to bring your body back into balance, and your eating and weight back under control.

TROUBLE TAMER: DAY #1

If you are having difficulty getting yourself to add low-carb protein to every meal and snack, you may be shortchanging yourself on the time needed to put yourself first. Are you placing the needs of your family, friends, children, even your pets ahead of your own? Then you probably need the motivation that our chapter on Healthy Selfishness can provide. All of the recipes, tips, and tactics in the world won't mean a thing if you never get a chance to take advantage of them. You need a crash course in how to get some essential *Me Time*. Read Chapter 2 and reread it until you can make space in your life for your own dreams and your own weight-loss success.

Move to Day #2 within a day or two, as you continue to add protein to each meal and snack.

THE 7-DAY JUMP-START PLAN

FOODS HIGH IN SATURATED FAT MAY INCREASE INSULIN
LEVELS AND CRAVINGS AND MAY SLOW WEIGHT LOSS.
ALWAYS TRY TO CHOOSE PROTEINS THAT ARE LOW IN
FAT FOR YOUR HEALTH'S SAKE AND WEIGHT LOSS TOO.

MEATS:

ALL REGULAR AND LEAN MEATS
INCLUDING:

Bacon
Beef
Ham
Hamburger
Hot dogs (that contain no
  added sugars or fillers)
Lamb
Pork
Rabbit
Sausages (that contain no
  added sugars or fillers)
Veal
Venison

FISH AND SHELLFISH:

ALL VARIETIES, CANNED, JARRED
(NO SUGAR), OR COOKED (NO
BREADING):

Bass	Perch
Bluefish	Salmon
Calamari	Sardines
Clams	Scallops
Cod	Scrod
Crabmeat	Shrimp
Flounder	Smelt
Haddock	Sole
Halibut	Sturgeon
Lobster	Swordfish
Monkfish	Trout
Oysters	Tuna

---

*Low-carb protein choices should comply with your physician's recommendations regarding dietary fat intake. (See page 115 to discover which cuts of your favorite meat are lowest in saturated fat.)

LOW-CARB PROTEIN LIST*

IMPORTANT NOTE: WHILE FOLLOWING THIS PLAN, IF A
PROTEIN IS NOT LISTED ON THESE TWO PAGES,
DO NOT CONSIDER IT TO BE LOW-CARB.

FOWL:

LIGHT OR DARK VARIETIES, WITH
OR WITHOUT SKIN, INCLUDING:

Capon
Chicken
Cornish hen
Duck
Goose
Luncheon meats (sliced
    chicken or turkey
    breast) (that contain no
    added sugars or fillers)
Pheasant
Quail
Squab
Turkey (ground or whole)

DAIRY AND NON-MEAT ALTERNATIVES:

REGULAR OR LOW-FAT
VARIETIES OF:

Cheese (all varieties,
    low-fat or regular)
Cottage cheese
Cream cheese
Eggs
Egg whites
Milk, cream, or half-and-
    half (use sparingly in
    coffee or tea; no
    nondairy creamers)
Sour cream
Tofu (soybean curd)*

---

*If you are particularly sensitive to monosodium glutamate, you may find that tofu can cause increased hunger, cravings, or reduced weight loss. If so, or if you are concerned, eliminate it from all meals.

Chapter 5

DAY #2: BACK IN CONTROL

GUIDELINE: ADD ON LOW-CARB VEGETABLES AND/OR SALAD TO LUNCH, DINNER, AND SNACKS.

Continue to follow the Guideline from Day #1.

The fiber found in vegetables can help stabilize your blood sugar levels. When fiber gets a chance to combine with protein, the positive effects are multiplied. Good fiber and low-carb protein eaten together can help stabilize blood sugars throughout the day, which can translate into more energy, clearer thinking, better motivation, fewer mood swings, and, of course, a drop in carbohydrate cravings.

To maximize the effects of the low-carb protein you've started to add to your meals and snacks, on Day #2 add some low-carb vegetables that are packed with fiber. Remember to continue eating the low-carb protein with each meal and snack as you did on Day #1, but now add some vegetables and/or salad to each meal or snack as well.

For Day #2's meals, choose from any of the low-carb vegetables or salad makings listed on the 7-Day Jump-Start Plan Low-Carb Vegetable and Salad List on page 53. Add at least one vegetable or salad to each meal or snack, and continue to add low-carb protein.

Some of the "low-carb" vegetables on low-carb lists you have used in the past may actually be high in carbohydrates (causing cravings and interfering with weight loss).

For now, use the low-carb vegetable list in this book only!

Do not use food lists from previous diets while following this plan (even if the lists say that they are low-carb). Some vegetable and salad makings that may have been included in other programs may actually be too high in carbohydrates for your particular metabolic profile. (For more info, see the "Hidden Carbs" chapter in this book.)

Using only the 7-Day Jump-Start Plan Low-Carb Vegetable and Salad List on page 53 as a guide, include at least one vegetable and/or salad in lunch, dinner, and every snack you eat today.

Whenever you can, and in keeping with your physician's recommendations, make sure the vegetables and/or salad you add *taste good*. Do not, we repeat do *not*, attempt to force down a mountain of mushy vegetables boiled to death and boring to eat. No matter how motivated you are, you can only put up with so much for so long. So to your dinner add some asparagus with a delicious hollandaise sauce (or low-fat cheese), or stuffed mushrooms. For each lunch or snack, enjoy an appetizing stir-fry, a curried chicken salad, or some cream-cheese stuffed celery.*

The amount of vegetables and salad that you add is not as important as being consistent—add them at each lunch, dinner, and snack as requested by that day's Guideline.

If you can and are willing to do so, the addition of one full "average" serving of vegetables and/or salad to every lunch, din-

---

*You'll find a wide variety of suggestions in the "Rescue Recipes" chapter of this book as well as in our *Carbohydrate Addict's Cookbook.*

ner, and snack is ideal. Adding two different vegetables or a vegetable and a salad to the same meal is a great way to be sure of getting a good fiber supplement.

Let's see how the Guideline for Day #2 plays out in real life. But first, a clarification: for purposes of illustration and to best explain how to incorporate the 7-Day Jump-Start Plan into your daily eating, we give examples using the same foods each day. In this way, we can best show how a meal changes throughout the Plan according to each day's Guidelines. The meals we describe in our examples are used as illustrations only, and because of that, they don't vary from day to day. You, on the other hand, should choose from a wide variety of low-carb vegetables, salad makings, and proteins.

So here we are at Day #2 and it's time for breakfast. Although, originally, you would have had only a bagel with cream cheese, in keeping with yesterday's Guideline of adding low-carb protein to every meal, you have now added some scrambled eggs.

You don't need to do anything at breakfast because Day #2's Guideline requires the addition of fiber only to lunches, dinners, and snacks. So just continue following Day #1's Guideline for that meal. If you want to add a salad or some vegetables to breakfast, that would be a welcome addition, but it is not necessary.

For lunch, dinner, and snacks today, however, the addition of one or more vegetables and/or a salad is required. Here's how a typical meal might play out: imagine that you're planning your favorite dinner at a restaurant—a shrimp appetizer, garlic bread, spaghetti with sauce, three or four meatballs, and a glass of wine. This meal contains a portion of low-carb protein as described in Day #1's Guideline (actually you've included two portions—even better), so you're all set to incorporate Day #2's Guideline of added low-carb vegetables.

Glancing over the 7-Day Jump-Start Plan Low-Carb Vegetable and Salad List on page 53, you decide to add both a low-carb vegetable and a salad to your dinner. So when ordering your meal, you also ask for a Caesar salad and a side order of asparagus. With these additions, you've met Day #2's Guidelines perfectly.

Here's how a sample day might look:

DAY #2 EXAMPLES

Old ***Breakfast Using*** ***Prior Guideline***	*New* ***Day #2*** ***Breakfast***
1–2 SCRAMBLED EGGS* BAGEL WITH CREAM CHEESE COFFEE WITH MILK	1–2 SCRAMBLED EGGS* BAGEL WITH CREAM CHEESE COFFEE WITH MILK (No change needed)
Old ***Lunch Using*** ***Prior Guideline***	*New* ***Day #2*** ***Lunch***
CHICKEN NOODLE SOUP ROLL AND BUTTER ¼ ROTISSERIE CHICKEN COKE LARGE CHOCOLATE CHIP COOKIE	CHICKEN NOODLE SOUP ROLL AND BUTTER ¼ ROTISSERIE CHICKEN COKE LARGE CHOCOLATE CHIP COOKIE *ADD* SIDE SALAD (LETTUCE, MUSHROOMS, GREEN PEPPERS, AND CUCUMBER) WITH BUTTERMILK DRESSING (See Recipe Chapter)

---

*Or the equivalent in egg whites or egg substitute.

Old Dinner Using Prior Guideline	*New Day #2 Dinner*
SHRIMP DIJON APPETIZER (See Recipe Chapter)	SHRIMP DIJON APPETIZER (See Recipe Chapter)
GARLIC BREAD	GARLIC BREAD
SPAGHETTI WITH SAUCE	SPAGHETTI WITH SAUCE
3–4 MEATBALLS	3–4 MEATBALLS
GLASS OF WINE	GLASS OF WINE
PLATE OF FRESH FRUIT	PLATE OF FRESH FRUIT
	ADD
	CAESAR SALAD
	AND
	ASPARAGUS (FEW SPEARS)
Old Late-Night Snack Using Prior Guideline	*New Day #2 Late-Night Snack*
3–4 BUFFALO CHICKEN DRUMETTES	3–4 BUFFALO CHICKEN DRUMETTES
POTATO CHIPS	POTATO CHIPS
CHOCOLATE BAR	CHOCOLATE BAR
	ADD
	CUCUMBER SLICES AND CELERY STICKS
	OR
	SMALL SALAD

On Day #2, as you begin adding vegetables and salad to your lunch, dinner, and snacks, you may be keenly aware of eating more food than you're used to. A snack may begin to look like a small meal. Remember that the quantity of low-carb vegetables and salad you add is up to you. Ideally, you will add an "average" portion, similar to that which you would get in a restaurant, but if you prefer, you can add less. If you are enjoying the vegetables and salad and *naturally* want to reduce your carbohydrate intake for that meal or snack—*not* because you have to, but because you *want* to—feel free to leave a bit of your carbo-hydrate-rich food on your plate.

As in Day #1, you may be surprised at how quickly your cravings for carbohydrate-rich foods drop as the power of fiber combines with low-carb protein to help balance your blood sugar levels. Remember: no matter how much carbohydrate you are including in your meals and snacks, add *some* vegetables or a salad to your plate along with your low-carb protein at every lunch, dinner, and snack.

> There is almost nothing more demoralizing
> than facing yet another mound of
> unappetizing, unadorned vegetables.
> We won't let you do it.

What should you do if you are already eating a good portion of vegetables and/or salad at a meal? Unless your physician rec-ommends otherwise, add a second portion. A second vegetable or a larger salad can help to further decrease your need for car-bohydrates, which, in turn, can help you lose weight more quickly and effortlessly.

Never Again

There is almost nothing more demoralizing than facing yet an-other mound of unappetizing, unadorned vegetables. We won't let you do it! You've got to choose a wide variety of raw and cooked vegetables (as always, in keeping with your physician's recommendations) and mix and match veggies whenever possi-ble. We love to stir-fry some green beans in olive oil and add whatever raw low-carb vegetables are handy: celery, green pep-per, cauliflower, and especially, mushrooms. Raw celery stuffed with cream cheese can easily be kept in the fridge for a quick addition to any snack, and topping a salad with some cheese shavings and sautéed chopped beef turns a bunch of lettuce into a taco salad.

The more high-fiber foods you add, the better for your program. And the more variety and better tasting the vegetables and salad that are available to you, the more of them you'll eat. Check out the "TroubleShooting" chapter in this book for simple tips on how to keep vegetables and salad makings at your fingertips, without letting food preparation take a bite out of your day. As a backup, you always have our "Rescue Recipes" in your corner. Check out that chapter for good starting ideas and emergency solutions. For other easy and exciting low-carb vegetable dishes and salad, choose among the many quick and easy choices in our *Carbohydrate Addict's Cookbook,* or any other low-carb cookbook that you are certain includes only low-carb ingredients.

Adding vegetables and salad to your regular eating program is like making any other change. It takes a little bit of energy at first, but if you do it *your* way, selecting those choices that best suit your tastes and needs, and listen to your own preferences ("I'd be willing to eat vegetables if I can put cheese on them" or "I hate boiled vegetables but I can handle them stir-fried" or "I won't eat salad plain but put my favorite dressing on it and I'll eat a mountain of it"), you'll find yourself moving toward a program that is far more likely to help you become successful and stay successful.

A Word Of Advice For The Veggie Hater

On occasion, we come across someone who says that they simply hate vegetables. "All vegetables?" we ask. "All vegetables!" they confirm. On further questioning, however, we usually discover that there are at least one or two low-carb vegetables they can tolerate, even if they don't actually enjoy them.

Once you're open to even one vegetable, you can begin to experiment with various ways of preparing it that might make it more interesting to you. And once you hit on a particularly appealing method (or two) of preparation, you might be open to trying that method with another vegetable. By gradually building upon a vegetable repertoire in this way, we've found that most people eventually come up with enough variety to make the program work for them.

Still not convinced? Then the following story might change your mind.

Anything But Vegetables: Alex's Story

There are some people whom you immediately like. Alex was one of those amazingly *likable* guys. Both Richard and I smile whenever we think of him. Standing a good six feet, six inches and weighing over three hundred pounds, Alex was hardly the kind of person who would fade into the background. But it was not his size that made you notice Alex (or Sasha as we came to call him, per his family's distant Russian royal connection). Part of what made Alex special was his smile and his twinkling eyes and the unwavering conviction with which he expressed his opinions—of the moment.

> "Don't ask me to eat vegetables."

"I'll do anything but just don't ask me to eat vegetables," Alex explained. "I *can't* balance my meals with fiber. It simply isn't going to happen—not now, not ever—and if that's what it's going to take for me to lose weight, then I'm going to have to stay fat for the rest of my life."

Crossing his arms over his great frame, Alex looked more like a frustrated five-year-old than one of New York's top trial lawyers. It took all we could muster to keep from smiling. We were certain that his problem wasn't half as bad as he thought it was. We also knew that he wouldn't believe us; at least, not at first.

Slowly, we began to explore Alex's history, gathering the information we needed to try and help. As a child, Alex had been forced to eat vegetables—tasteless mounds of mush. His father, himself an overworked and underachieving lawyer, had used young Alex's distaste for vegetables (if you could call them that) as a topic of argument and control, often sending Alex to bed—mid-meal—if the boy would not eat as his father directed. The man had been huge, greater in bulk that his son was now, and had often resorted to physical abuse in retribution for Alex's terrible crime of refusing to eat vegetables.

"I know, of course, it had nothing to do with me," Alex explained. "My father was unable to think on his feet in court, though he thought well enough when it came to calling me names and threatening me. He should never have been a trial lawyer," Alex concluded with a sad shake of his head. "Maybe then I'd be thin," he added with a wry smile.

Alex hadn't eaten anything green
for twenty-five years.

Though he joked about it, we saw no humor in Alex's pain and we wouldn't allow him to dismiss it so easily. Although he was back to being his good-natured self, we helped Alex remember many of the incidents in which food in general, and vegetables in particular, preceded disapproval and punishment in his life. The wounds ran so deep that Alex confessed he had not eaten anything green since the day he left his parents' home twenty-five years earlier.

"Except for my sister-in-law's corned beef, and it was green 'cause it had been left outside at the pool party too long," he added with a grin.

Alex had lost weight on a low-carb diet but had not been eating any vegetables at all.

"I knew I couldn't keep it up, but I didn't know what else

to do," he added. "I want to go back on the diet as soon as you help me work up some of my self-control again."

We explained that we could not help him to return to so imbalanced an eating plan.

We were at an impasse.

Finally, we came to a compromise. In Alex's case, the vegetables that he had been forced to eat had been boiled to death. He might not have had a love of vegetables to start with, but given the way they had been prepared, coupled with the trauma of his father's fury, it was no wonder that he had developed a veggie-phobia.

It had been our experience, we explained, that no matter how much someone *thought* they hated vegetables, we were usually able to find *some* form of low-carb vegetable that they could enjoy. Okay, we agreed, *enjoy* might be too strong a word in his case; *tolerate* might be a better description, but in any case, if he would give us a chance, we thought we could come up with a solution that would allow him to eat more healthfully without making him want to gag.

He agreed. Barely. "I'll try on one condition," Alex added, with a teasing look. "No okra!"

We agreed and, after much prodding, discovered that there was, indeed, one vegetable that Alex actually liked. "My aunt makes this creamed spinach," he told us. "It's really not bad."

Behind the "not bad" was this story: every Thanksgiving, his aunt was sure to include her famous creamed spinach; in fact, she made Alex his own special casserole dish, filled to the top with the creamy mixture. Gratified by his enjoyment of her trademark dish, his aunt always made extra for Alex to take home with him.

"It's good cold too," Alex reported. "I have it with chips, you know, like a dip."

We had hit pay dirt! While Alex considered his dislike of vegetables to be a mere nuisance, we knew the importance of these foods in his long-term prospects for maintaining good health and an ideal weight. And now we had a starting point.

Since Alex was adamant about the fact that he didn't like creamed spinach prepared in any way other than according to his aunt's unique recipe, we began at the source.

On Alex's request, his aunt faxed us a copy of her recipe (and several other recipes she thought we might enjoy!). As we had hoped, her recipe was made almost entirely of low-carb ingredients. It was simple and quick and, more importantly, it supplied the fiber that Alex needed.

The creamed spinach recipe also gave us an important clue for shaping an eating program to Alex's taste. (If you're going to change your eating habits for life, you've got to be sure to tailor it to your own individual preferences and needs.) The creamed spinach that had won Alex's heart was spicy in the extreme!

No wonder he couldn't stick with a diet!
When he left the carbs behind,
he left the flavor behind as well.

That fact alone led us to discover that Alex liked—no, required—any food to be, as he put it, "full of taste." Looking at each of the times he had failed to stick to a low-carb diet in the past, we realized it was the "lack of flavor" that drove him back to his old way of eating. And no wonder. When Alex left the carbs behind, he left the flavor behind as well.

Divorced and living alone, he never cooked for himself. Whenever he attempted another stab at his old low-carb diet, he abandoned his favorite restaurants—the ones that made the best hot dishes in town. Instead of relishing a pile of enchiladas from Enrique's, Alex forced down a bland piece of poached fish at the local diner. Trading in his favorite curry dish complete with saffron rice and several side dishes of fried Indian bread in exchange for a dry slice of meatloaf may have helped in the weight-loss department, but it did not provide a pleasurable eating program on which he could live for life. Together, we worked out a strategy that succeeded not only for Alex but for thousands of others who followed him.

Here's how it works: If you think you don't like vegetables (or are certain of that fact), imagine any low-carb vegetable dish or salad ingredient that you are willing to try. Figure out what it is about that dish that makes it more palatable than others. If it is the type of vegetable, start being inventive! Cream it, sauté it, stir-fry it, make it the basis of a casserole or soufflé by combining it with low-carb protein, or simply top it with low-fat cheese. Use your vegetable in any recipe you can imagine. Take any low-carb vegetable recipe and substitute your vegetable for the vegetable listed in the ingredients. Voilà! You've multiplied your vegetable intake by ten.

You can't be expected
to eat the same old vegetables every day.

Be as inventive as you like. (Richard loves sautéed green peppers cold, though I can barely stand to watch him eat them.) Find whatever pleases you. Just remember, whatever you do, don't ask yourself to eat the same old plain, steamed, overcooked vegetables every day. You won't. And you shouldn't be expected to.

If you only like your vegetable or salad ingredient raw, consider adding a wide variety of low-carb dips, salad dressings, and toppings. There are many that fit the low-carb profile and they can make all the difference in the world. You'll find a variety of fun suggestions in our "Rescue Recipes" chapter. Gradually begin to substitute other vegetables, starting with the ones you like best (or, at least, those you are willing to eat). As you add new vegetables, always remember to keep the key ingredients you liked best in that first, favorite recipe. You might move from a spinach soufflé, for instance, to an asparagus soufflé, changing only the type of vegetable. From there, you might try asparagus topped with the same cheese you liked in the soufflé, and so on.

Alex took on the challenge of putting the spice back in his life. Returning to his favorite restaurants, he worked out low-carb meals that would help him lose weight without losing the joy of eating.

Once he realized that adding fiber didn't mean eating sawdust or overcooked "mush," the change in Alex was astounding. Not only did he figure out how to get far more satisfying low-carb choices at his favorite restaurants, he also began to cook, a first for him! We started him out with his aunt's formula for creamed spinach and gave him our own recipe for crustless quiche, which we enhanced with a spicy addition just for him. (You'll find it in our Rescue Recipe chapter).

He loved the idea that he could make two or three quiches, cut them into meal-sized portions, freeze them, and whenever he wanted, thaw a wedge and eat it at room temperature or reheat it in the microwave.

Once he started, Alex became a fireball on his own. In a matter of weeks, he had worked out a palette of spicy Indian, Mexican, Brazilian, and Greek recipes—all made with a variety of low-carb vegetables and each more delicious than the other. Like our quiche, he made them in batches and froze them in serving sizes (which he said were getting smaller without any effort on his part). When he needed them, they were there waiting; a few minutes in the microwave and he had legal veggies that actually tasted good!

Rather than going back to his old low-carb program, Alex decided to move into our Carbohydrate Addict's LifeSpan Program. Being able to enjoy the high-carb foods he loved once a day in a Reward Meal®, along with low-carb meals that cut his cravings and the weight, made the entire experience a lot more fun.

His low-carb meals included so wide a variety of dishes that he took up cooking as a hobby and often uses his vacation time to enroll in a "cook's tour class."

Down more than sixty-five pounds for almost five years now, Alex called the other day to say hello and to share an important insight.

"I think I understand my father's hang-up with vegetables," he explained. "It came to me yesterday. I was looking in the mirror, wishing my father could have seen me the way I look now, and I realized how frustrated he must have been with his own weight. His own father had been huge and my father must have been afraid I would end up just like him."

There was a pause. We waited.

"In his own way," Alex continued quietly, "he was trying to save me from the same fate, but he just didn't know how."

We are proud of Alex and very happy for him. He has opened himself up to new experiences with food, and in doing so, he has broken a cycle of pain and anger that had spanned two generations.

TROUBLE TAMER: DAY #2

If adding low-carb vegetables and/or salad to your meals and snacks proves to be a challenge, you may need to spend a day or two with this Guideline until you feel that you have conquered it. Don't move on until you can imagine a variety of low-carb vegetables and/or salads that you would find appealing as part of your regular eating program.

If you hate vegetables (in general), it's essential that you make low-carb vegetables and/or salad a pleasurable experience by starting with one or two vegetables and expanding your horizons. Use some of the recipes in this book, in our *Carbohydrate Addict's Cookbook*, or in any other low-carb cookbook that is certain to include only low-carb ingredients. If you can't even imagine the words "vegetables" and "salad" in the same sentence as "pleasurable," put some energy into this essential part of any lifetime lifestyle change. From stuffed mushrooms to

Alex's New Orleans Quiche, we know you'll find a few recipes that will provide some good fiber first aid.

Move to Day #3 in a day or two, as soon as you've roped in a fair number of low-carb vegetable and salad alternatives that you can live with, enjoy, and add to your lunches, dinners, and snacks.

THE 7-DAY JUMP-START PLAN
LOW-CARB VEGETABLE AND SALAD LIST

IMPORTANT NOTE: WHILE FOLLOWING THIS PLAN, IF A VEGETABLE OR SALAD INGREDIENT IS NOT LISTED BELOW, DO NOT CONSIDER IT TO BE LOW-CARB.

VEGETABLE AND SALAD MAKINGS:
RAW, STIR-FRIED, SAUTÉED (NO BREADING ADDED), STEAMED, OR BOILED NON-STARCHY VEGETABLES:

Alfalfa sprouts	Kale
Arugula	Kohlrabi
Asparagus	Lettuce
Bamboo shoots	Mushrooms
Bean sprouts	Okra
Bok Choy	Parsley
Brussels sprouts	Peppers (green only)
Cabbage (all)	Radishes
Cauliflower	Scallions
Celery	Snap beans
Cucumbers	Sorrel
Endive	Sour grass
Green beans	Spinach
Greens (all)	Wax beans

Chapter 6

DAY #3: BALANCED AGAIN

GUIDELINE: BALANCE ALL MEALS AND SNACKS.

Include a good portion of low-carb protein, vegetables, and/or salad in relation to high-carb foods. Continue both prior guidelines.

This Guideline can help increase weight loss and cut cravings by using a simple strategy that works with your body's natural response to lower-carbohydrate foods. On Day #1 and Day #2 you were asked to include "some" low-carb protein or low-carb vegetable or salad. While you were encouraged to include an "average serving," that is, the size of a portion you might get at a restaurant, you weren't required to do so. If you have been including only a few bites of low-carb food at meals or snacks, here's your chance to better balance your eating and better balance your blood sugar and insulin levels as well.

Today's Guideline requests that you use the amount of protein in a meal to determine the maximum amount of high-carbohydrate food you will eat at that same meal. In that way, you are balancing the quantity of the carbohydrates with an equal quantity of low-carb protein. You don't need to weigh or measure anything; just use your eye to make sure that you're not over-carbing.

We'll go over the details in the coming pages, but here's a

quick overview: To get a good balance, for breakfast the portions can be divided up to half high-carb foods and half low-carb protein. You can eat more low-carb protein than high-carb foods but never more high-carb than low-carb. With your physician's approval, you can choose to eat all low-carb protein, and if you like, you can add low-carb vegetables and salad makings to your breakfast. High fiber is a welcome addition as long as you make certain not to eat more high-carb foods than you eat of low-carb protein.

At lunch, dinner, and snacks, continue the same balance: eat only as much high-carb food (including starches and sweets in total) as you eat of low-carb protein at that meal. Again, you may choose to eat more low-carb protein than high-carb foods but never the reverse.

At lunch, dinner, and snacks you should also include at least as much low-carb vegetables and/or salad as low-carb protein. If you would like to eat a greater quantity of veggies and salad, that would be excellent, but if that's not your preference, at least eat an equal quantity of low-carb veggies/salad as you eat of low-carb protein. In other words, at most, one-third of your meal should be made up of carbohydrate-rich foods along with one-third low-carb protein and one-third low-carb vegetable and/or salad.

To enhance your insulin and blood sugar balance and to speed up your weight loss and cut cravings, you can choose to eat a smaller quantity of high-carbohydrate foods than your portion of low-carb protein, but don't push yourself to the point of feeling deprived.

The balance of low-carb protein and
low-carb vegetables to high–carb
foods is very important.

You may already have noticed that you feel
"better" when you eat enough protein and
vegetables to balance the high-carb foods.

A Question Of Quantity

We want to make sure it's clear that in order to meet Guideline #3 you never need to weigh or measure your food and you most certainly do not have to count carb grams. At each meal, simply consider carbohydrate-rich foods as well as the low-carb protein and low-carb vegetable and/or salad you will be including in your meal and make certain that your total intake of high-carb food does not exceed your intake of low-carb protein. In addition, at lunch, dinner, and snacks, match the amount of the low-carb vegetables and/or salad you eat to your low-carb protein as well.

The balance of low-carb protein and low-carb vegetables and salad with respect to high–carb foods is very important. If you shift your meals in the high-carb direction too much or too often, you may not get the full craving and weight-reducing benefits of your low-carb protein and fiber. Blood sugar and insulin levels will almost certainly go out of kilter. Balance in enough low-carb protein and low-carb veggies, on the other hand, and the effect is amazing.

In our first book, *The Carbohydrate Addict's Diet,* we explained that the Reward Meal—that is, the single daily meal in which you get to enjoy carbohydrate-rich foods while still maintaining a low-carb profile for the rest of the day—should be "balanced," and not a binge. That is, the Reward Meal should include low-carb protein and vegetables as well as carbohydrate-rich foods. We encouraged our readers to choose from a variety of foods, and we explained that insulin's impact was usually the underlying cause of recurring cravings and the tendency to gain weight easily. Most of all, we (repeatedly) stressed the importance of balancing all carbohydrate-rich foods with low-carb protein and fiber-filled vegetables and/or salads.

Unfortunately, when this book became a *New York Times* bestseller, the media, anxious to have something controversial and sensational to say about it, interpreted "balanced" as some sort of frenzied food free-for-all. We could never figure that one out! Contrary to everything we had actually written, the media was attributing to our plan menus that were so carbohydrate loaded as to sink a ship!

There was nothing we could do to stop the flow of misinformation. I remember looking at one grocery store tabloid that claimed to show a week's meal plan that conformed with our guidelines. Richard looked at the terribly out-of-balance menus and commented, "I don't know whose diet this is, but it certainly isn't ours!"

Several years later, in our newer book *The Carbohydrate Addict's LifeSpan Program,* we were able to carefully define the ideal balance of the Reward Meal. *The Carbohydrate Addict's LifeSpan Program* hit #1 on the *New York Times* bestseller list, and it conveyed information that few reporters could easily distort. Readers, old and new alike, were able to make the best choices possible in order to get the greatest benefit from our program.

Below, we've included a detailed description that will help you meet Day #3's Guideline of balance, balance, balance.

On this plan you never have to weigh,
measure, or count carbs.
Most people simply can't live by the
"numbers" (nor do they *want* to).

Balance Made Easy

Breakfast: Balance your meal so that the amount of carbohydrate-rich food you eat is not greater than the amount of low-carb protein you consume at that meal. If you are also choosing to include low-carb salad and/or vegetables in your breakfast, consider that an added benefit but still make certain your high-carb intake does not exceed your low-carb protein intake. You may choose all low-carb protein, or mostly low-carb protein along with some high-carb, but in any case, eat no more high-carb food than you eat of low-carb protein.

BREAKFAST BALANCE:

FOR EACH PORTION OF LOW-CARB PROTEIN . . .

(that is, regular or low-fat varieties of meats, poultry, fish, cheese, eggs, and tofu in our Low-Carb Protein List on page 36)

INCLUDE *NO MORE* THAN AN EQUAL PORTION OF CARBOHYDRATE-RICH FOODS.

(including starches such as breads, pasta, rice, etc.; starchy vegetables such as potatoes, peas, corn, carrots, etc.; snack foods, fruits, juices, and sweets)

THEREFORE, AT BREAKFAST, YOUR PORTION OF HIGH-CARB FOODS SHOULD *NOT* BE GREATER THAN THAT OF YOUR LOW-CARB PROTEIN (ALTHOUGH YOU MAY HAVE AS FEW HIGH-CARB FOODS AS YOU LIKE).

In addition, if you desire them at breakfast, you can include all of the low-carb vegetables and/or salad you wish from our Low-Carb Vegetable and Salad List (page 53). While these high-fiber foods are very good for you, and may speed your weight loss and bring about a greater reduction in cravings, they are not required at breakfast.

Lunch, Dinner, and Snacks: Balance these meals and snacks so that at lunch, dinner, or snack, your low-carb protein and low-carb vegetable and/or salad portions are about equal. In addition, make certain that your high-carb portion is never greater than *either* your low-carb protein or low-carb vegetable portion.

In other words, *at most*, about one-third of your meal should be made up of carbohydrate-rich foods along with one-third low-carb protein and one-third low-carb vegetable and/or salad. You may decide to have a minimal amount of high-carb foods at a meal and concentrate mainly on low-carb protein and low-carb vegetables and/or salad. Or you may include no high-carb foods at all, including only low-carb protein and low-carb vegetables and/or salad in a meal. That's your choice. The balance requirement here is, first, that the amount of your low-carb protein be equal to the amount of your low-carb vegetables and/or salad and, second, that the amount of high-carb food you include in that meal is equal to or less than your portion of low-carb protein.

LUNCH, DINNER, AND SNACK BALANCE:
FOR EACH PORTION OF LOW-CARB PROTEIN . . .
(that is, regular or low-fat varieties of meats, poultry, fish, cheese, eggs, and tofu in our Low-Carb Protein List on page 36)

INCLUDE AN EQUAL AMOUNT OF LOW-CARB
VEGETABLES AND/OR SALAD . . .
(including non-starchy vegetables as listed in our Low-Carb Vegetable and Salad List on page 53)

AND, IF YOU LIKE, A PORTION OF CARBOHYDRATE-RICH FOODS . . .
(including starches such as breads, pasta, rice, etc.; starchy vegetables such as potatoes, peas, corn, carrots, etc.; snack foods, fruits, juices, and sweets)
THAT IS EQUAL TO *NO MORE* THAN YOUR PORTION
OF LOW-CARB PROTEIN.

THEREFORE, AT LUNCH, DINNER, AND SNACKS, YOUR PORTION OF HIGH-CARB FOODS SHOULD *NOT* BE GREATER THAN ONE-THIRD OF THE MEAL (ALTHOUGH IT CAN BE AS LITTLE AS YOU LIKE).

In The Eye Of The Beholder

Remember, on this plan you will never be asked to weigh, measure, or count carbs. (How long could anyone be expected to live by the "numbers"?) In order to balance your meal, simply eyeball your portions and, of course, use your good judgment. If you are including a small portion of roast beef (low-carb protein) and want some baked potato (high-carb), include a portion of potato about equal in size to the meat as it will look on your plate. If you want bread and baked potato (both high-carb), take smaller portions so that the total portion equals that of your low-carb protein (or, if you prefer, increase your portion of protein a bit).

A Word Of Caution

Do not choose a portion of protein that is too much for you to eat just so you can eat a greater quantity of high-carb food and still meet the Guideline for Day #3. Make choices that are in keeping with the Guideline. And one last thought: do not pile up the protein, add on the high-carb foods, then eat the high-carbs but leave the protein on your plate. That is not the deal!

As Far As The Protein Will Stretch

Sometimes balance just isn't enough. At Day #3, you may find that one or more of your meals is just so carbo-loaded, it would take more low-carb protein and low-carb veggies and/or salad to balance it out than would be wise to eat. If this is the case, your only choices are to eat *very* small portions of the several high-carb foods you want to include in that meal or, a far better choice, select one or two high-carbohydrate foods and balance this far more reasonable meal with low-carb protein, vegetables, and/or salad. Remember than no one is asking you to give up these foods forever. Right now, we're only pointing out that saving them for another meal might allow you to eat your cake and lose weight too.

DAY #3 EXAMPLES

Note: If a meal is very carb heavy (as in lunch in the following example), the addition of one or more low-carb proteins and low-carb salads and vegetables to make a better balance, as explained in today's Guideline, could result in a meal that is simply too large for reasonable comfort and good sense. If a meal has become too large because of the added balance of low-carb protein and low-carb vegetables and/or salad, either (1) cut down on the size of the portions of all foods in that meal (low-carb and high-carb alike) or (2) cut the amount of only the carbohydrate-rich foods in that meal.

DAY #3 EXAMPLES

Old *Breakfast Using* *Prior Guidelines*	*New* *Day #3* *Breakfast*
1–2 SCRAMBLED EGGS* BAGEL WITH CREAM CHEESE COFFEE WITH MILK	2 SCRAMBLED EGGS* A SMALL BAGEL WITH CREAM CHEESE COFFEE WITH MILK (Portions increased or cut in size for balance)
Old *Lunch Using* *Prior Guidelines*	*New* *Day #3* *Lunch*
CHICKEN NOODLE SOUP ROLL AND BUTTER SIDE SALAD WITH BUTTERMILK DRESSING (See Recipe Chapter) ¼ ROTISSERIE CHICKEN COKE LARGE CHOCOLATE CHIP COOKIE	(REMOVED CHICKEN NOODLE SOUP FOR BALANCE)† SMALL ROLL AND BUTTER LARGE SALAD WITH BUTTERMILK DRESSING (See Recipe Chapter) ½ ROTISSERIE CHICKEN SMALL COKE ½ LARGE CHOCOLATE CHIP COOKIE (Portions increased or cut in size for balance)

*Or the equivalent in egg whites or a cheese omelet, preferably low-fat.

†Even after balancing, this meal remained too high-carb heavy. To balance, we removed high-carb food.

Old *Dinner Using* *Prior Guidelines*	*New* *Day #3* *Dinner*
CAESAR SALAD SHRIMP DIJON APPETIZER (See Recipe Chapter) GARLIC BREAD SPAGHETTI WITH SAUCE 3–4 MEATBALLS ASPARAGUS GLASS OF WINE PLATE OF FRESH FRUIT	CAESAR SALAD SHRIMP DIJON APPETIZER (See Recipe Chapter) SMALL GARLIC BREAD OR SIDE ORDER SPAGHETTI WITH SAUCE* 3–4 MEATBALLS ASPARAGUS GLASS OF WINE PLATE OF FRESH FRUIT (Portions increased or cut in size for balance)
Old *Late-Night Snack* *Using Prior Guidelines*	*New Day #3* *Late-Night* *Snack*
3–4 BUFFALO CHICKEN DRUMETTES CUCUMBER SLICES AND CELERY STICKS POTATO CHIPS CHOCOLATE BAR	6–8 BUFFALO CHICKEN DRUMETTES LARGE SIDE DISH OF CUCUMBER SLICES AND CELERY STICKS SMALL PORTION OF POTATO CHIPS SMALL CHOCOLATE BAR (Portions increased or cut in size for balance)

Ahead Of Your Time

It's possible that even before you came to Day #3's Guideline you already had a balanced intake of high-carb foods in comparison to your low-carb protein and low-carb vegetable and/or

---

*Even after balancing, this meal remained too high-carb heavy. In order to balance this meal, we removed one of the high-carb foods.

salad portions. In that case, you might already be meeting this Guideline.

If have read through Day #3's Guideline to make certain you understand all the details, *and* you find that you are already following this Guideline, then you have a choice. You can move on to Day #4 and begin to incorporate that day's Guideline, which will put you one day ahead of your Plan and that much closer to your goal of struggle-free weight loss. Or you can consider Day #3 to be a day in which you need to change nothing. It's really up to you. If you decide to change nothing today, remember to continue to balance your meals and snacks as you have been doing and enjoy the fact that you appear to be right on track. Whether you move on or stay put, in either case, you're doing beautifully.

TROUBLE TAMER: DAY #3

Perhaps you read and understood the concept of balance as described in the above Guideline, but when it came right down to it, you ate what you wanted. Or perhaps after reading over the Guideline once and finding that it required a bit of your attention, you decided that balance wasn't so important after all.

If these or any other reasons kept you from fully following Day #3's Guideline of balance, we would like you to consider the following: if you make the same choices over and over again, you will get the same results.

If you find it uncomfortable to reread something in order to fully grasp the fine details, or if you think you can mix and match recommendations from different diets with our Guidelines and still expect to be successful at losing weight and keeping it off, or if you just feel anxious when new ideas don't come easily and prefer to avoid them, we'd like you to gather up your resolve and fight your impulse to ignore Day #3's Guideline of balance.

Balancing your meals can make all the difference in the world. If you didn't succeed in balancing your meals today, keep trying for another day or two. Even if you'd prefer not to, reread this Guideline. (We have both discovered that when try-

ing to understand anything new, it helps to read it aloud to ourselves.) Plan the ways in which you can balance your meals,
and finally, take whatever steps are necessary to make it happen
(including demanding that your waiter bring your salad, now!).

Mark and Monique: Two Peas, Not of the Same Pod

From our first meeting, it was clear that Mark and Monique,
twenty-five-year-old twins, had their own, very distinct per-
sonalities. They were as opposite as any two people could
be. Mark had deep and intractable views on a variety of
subjects (and made that fact known from the start), while
Monique seemed to be open to new ideas and to the inter-
personal lifeline we were offering.

Mark, a senior lab technician, and Monique, a critical-care
nurse, had attended an in-service course we offered at New
York's Mount Sinai School of Medicine for nurses, physicians, and other health care professionals who wanted advice
on counseling their patients on low-carbohydrate dieting.

Following our lectures, Mark and Monique requested ap-
pointments with us to discuss their own personal battles
with eating and weight. We suggested that we see them together, assuming they might offer each other support. We
were sadly mistaken.

> They had tried "every diet in the world,"
> but their cravings and weight-loss plateaus
> usually made them lose motivation.

Over the course of several meetings, Mark argued every
fact we presented, including those for which he had little
background knowledge. Monique offered her thoughts but
clearly remained willing to try innovative ways of doing things.

"After all," she said in response to her brother's loudly voiced negative response to just about any help we had to offer, "what have I got to lose? Trying to do it on my own certainly hasn't been working."

Monique and Mark were each at least one hundred pounds over their ideal weight. Separately and together they had tried "every diet in the world," but their cravings and weight-loss plateaus usually made them lose their motivation within a short time. While low-carb dieting seemed to work for them for a while, their efforts always ended in failure. Both had gained back all the weight they had lost on low-carb diets . . . and more.

We gave them copies of our evolving 7-Day Jump-Start Plan, along with many other essential pieces of information and strategies that had proven repeatedly successful, and sent them off for two weeks on their own.

> "Most of all, I'm not *hungry*. It's amazing!
> I feel like I've got someone else's body
> . . . and I'm not giving it back."

Exactly fourteen days later, having completed the 7-Day Plan and spent an additional week putting into action the strategies, tips, and information we had given them, Monique and Mark returned to see us—but with decidedly different results.

Monique was ecstatic.

"Here's what I've been eating," she said, handing us her daily food log. "And here are my daily weights," she added proudly, handing us a second paper that showed in number (and graph!) her strong and steady weight loss.

"Most of all," she added with the same enthusiasm, "I'm not *hungry*. It's amazing! I feel like I've got someone else's body . . . and I'm not giving it back."

Mark's results were far less impressive. He brought in

food logs for only a few days and had weighed himself only sporadically. It was clear that he was not losing weight. He had experienced none of the drops in cravings that made his sister so happy, and although he had not given up, it seemed likely he would not stay on the program much longer.

Comparing their food logs, we confirmed what we had come to suspect in so many of the people who came to us for help. Monique had been following our suggestions to the letter. Her low-carb meals were free of high-carb foods and her Reward Meal choices were perfectly balanced. For every portion of bread, pasta, or dessert at Monique's Reward Meal, she had been careful to include an equal or greater portion of low-carb protein and low-carb vegetable.

When she wanted second helpings, a desire that Monique said was fading by the day, she made certain to take as much protein and low-carb vegetable as she did her high-carb choice.

"My dad took us all out to my favorite restaurant for their Sunday buffet," she said. "After eating my dinner and a piece of chocolate cake for dessert, and keeping the whole meal pretty well balanced, I decided to go back for seconds. I didn't really want it, and I certainly didn't need it, but I felt I had it coming to me. But instead of going back for just a piece of cake or two, I filled up a small plate with roast beef and asparagus and a second plate with cake.

> "By the time I got done,
> I didn't even *want* the cake."

"Now, here's what's crazy. By the time I finished my beef and asparagus—I didn't want the cake. I barely touched it. Even though I knew I was allowed to have it, I just didn't *feel* like it!"

Mark had gone along to the same buffet, but his experience

was quite the opposite, most likely because he had not "even thought" of balancing his high-carb food with lower-carb choices.

"I just wasn't in the mood," he admitted. "Besides, I just don't see how balancing could make any difference."

The results of that dinner's unbalanced meal should have proven the point to him, but it didn't. After loading up a plate with "several" crescent rolls and a large plate with pasta with marinara sauce, Mark bypassed the carving station (stocked with several cuts of turkey and prime rib) and headed for the table. His meal, virtually free of any significant protein or low-carb vegetables, was so imbalanced that after eating it, he "didn't feel the slightest bit" satisfied (although, as he put it, he was "stuffed").

"I felt full but not finished, you know?" he explained.

Returning to the buffet, Mark took seconds of the pasta and, still passing up the carving station, finished off a second helping. Fuller but still not satisfied, Mark hit the dessert bar, where he selected a slice of chocolate fudge cake and a crème brûlée. Finishing both desserts, he noticed Monique's uneaten cake and, since she had left it virtually untouched, asked if he could eat it.

"I couldn't get enough," Mark concluded. "And I was mad that she wouldn't give it to me though she clearly had no intention of eating it."

"That cake was mine!" Monique retorted. "Even if I didn't want to eat all of it, it made me happy just to see it sitting there, knowing I *could* have it if I wanted it."

Monique never did finish that second piece of cake or a thousand other second servings that she could have had.

In the months that followed, she moved into our Carbohydrate Addict's LifeSpan Program, in which she continued to enjoy one balanced Reward Meal each day along with low-carb meals and snacks, and incorporated other important changes to patterns of eating that had marked her downfall in the past.

Throughout those months, by giving special attention to balancing high-carbohydrate foods at her daily Reward Meal,

Monique was able to take off more than one hundred pounds. She has remained slim and healthy to this day, nearly a decade later.

> "I'd be happy to eat like this
> for the rest of my life," Monique told us
> at her first two-week check-in.
>
> One hundred pounds slimmer for almost
> ten years, she might very well do just that.

Mark, on the other hand, refused to even try to balance his meals. He has become heavier and, we're unhappy to report, unhealthier, with each passing year.

Their relationship is not as close now. Monique knows Mark resents her success, but he still remains "his same stubborn self," as she puts it. The harder she has tried to help him, the more critical Mark has become, until as far as he is concerned, there is virtually nothing his sister can do right. It seems such a waste to us, though we both know, too well, what it feels like to be left behind when others are losing weight and moving on with their lives.

In spite of Mark's negativity, Monique has made a wonderful life for herself. She married within a year of losing her weight and has twins of her own—two girls.

"I'd be happy to eat like this for the rest of my life," Monique told us so long ago at her first two-week check-in.

Now it seems she might very well do just that.

On a follow-up phone call, Monique told us that although she knew she was not to blame, she felt a bit guilty about "leaving Mark behind."

"I know it's his choice and he's just as stubborn as my father, but . . ."

We knew what she was having a hard time putting into words. It's difficult to feel you're leaving behind someone you love, even when they keep telling you to leave them alone. Perhaps someday . . .

For now, this is Monique's chance to enjoy the health, freedom, and family she has worked so hard and so long to attain. She has *earned* them!

Chapter 7

DAY #4: SAVING THE BEST FOR LAST

> **GUIDELINE:** AT ALL MEALS AND SNACKS, EAT *TOWARD* YOUR CARBS.
>
> Hold on until you've finished your low-carb protein, vegetables, and salad before you begin to eat your high-carb foods. Continue to follow all prior guidelines.

This is our favorite Guideline because it's so easy and it has such an immediate impact on how you feel. First, we need to explain why it succeeds so well; then we'll give you some easy ways to make this Guideline work for you.

When you eat too many carbohydrate-rich foods, or if you eat them too often, your body releases too much insulin. In time, the insulin can no longer enter cells as it normally should and becomes "trapped" in your bloodstream. Insulin is called the "hunger hormone" because of its power to make you crave carbohydrates. The more insulin in your bloodstream, the more powerful your craving for carbohydrates is likely to be.

> Insulin is called the "hunger hormone" because of its power to make you crave carbohydrates.

Most people know that an excellent way to reduce the amount of insulin trapped in your bloodstream, and to reduce your cravings and weight, is to eat fewer carbohydrate-rich foods. What few people realize is that another great way to reduce insulin levels in the blood is to shorten the amount of time that it takes you to consume these foods. The longer you linger over carbs, the higher your insulin level is likely to rise.

Chances are you've had the experience of eating until you were full, and then, for one reason or another, you continued to nibble at your dinner or dessert. It may have been a social situation where the conversation continued or where you were keeping someone company as they finished their meal. After continuing to eat past your satisfaction level, you might have noticed that you felt as if you could eat forever without feeling satisfied. In other words, you were less satisfied the longer you continued to eat. This example of "the longer I eat the less satisfied I feel" experience is due to the prolonged ability of insulin to block your body's stop-eating signal.

> Even when you just smell high-carb foods
> (like that microwaved popcorn),
> a flood of insulin makes you instantly hungry!

Insulin is released at two phases. When you see, smell, or taste carbohydrate-rich foods, the first flood of insulin is released and, suddenly, you're hungry. Ever smell microwaved popcorn and suddenly need to have some?

That first flood of insulin (or the smell, sight, or taste that signaled it) begins an Insulin Countdown. You now have about sixty minutes before a second release of insulin will occur, a failsafe mechanism that provides additional insulin your body might need as you eat more carbohydrates. If you continue to eat past sixty minutes, that second release of insulin will give your body a powerful message to keep eating.

For that reason, the Guideline for Day #4 requests that you eat *toward* your carbohydrates in every meal and snack. Start off eating your low-carb salad, vegetables, and protein, and finish them before you begin to eat your carbohydrate-rich foods, moving from the starchy foods to the sweets. (Fruit and fruit juices are considered sweets; save them until the end.)

Ideally, you will start to feel satisfied, even a bit full, before the starches and sweets ever enter your mouth. In that way, the amount of time insulin has to be released is greatly shortened and with it, your cravings. As an added bonus, less insulin can mean reduced insulin resistance; your body is able to burn up fat rather than store it.

> Restaurants know that the bread
> you eat at the beginning of a meal
> will make you order more food, even though
> you'll be too full to eat it all!

This Guideline may be like none you've ever seen or heard about, but the power of carbohydrate-rich foods to stimulate your hunger is well known. For example, restaurants, wanting you to order more food, give you bread right away. They know that once your body is flooded with insulin, you'll order more food (even if you're too stuffed to eat it by the time it comes). Traditional appetizers are typically high-carb for the same reason. (Why else would they be called appetizers?)

Once you get some practice, this Guideline will become a dear and valuable friend. It will allow you to enjoy the carbs you love while sidestepping some of insulin's powerful hunger and weight-gain effects.

To follow Day #4's Guideline, begin your meal or snack with the salad makings, vegetables, and protein portions you added in Day #1 and Day #2 (from the Low-Carb Protein and Low-Carb Vegetable lists in this book). Eat your low-carb protein and low-carb vegetables first, preferably until you feel begin to feel satisfied. Then begin to enjoy your more carbohydrate-rich foods, vegetables that are not included in our 7-Day Jump-Start Low-Carb Vegetable and Salad List (like carrots, peas, and potatoes), then the starches (including pasta and bread) and/or dessert, each time moving from the less starchy to the more starchy foods, and finally to the sweets, as your meal progresses.

Don't worry about being exact. You don't have to count carb grams. We have not included a chart or table because we want you to use your own experience and judgment. This Guideline is concerned with your *general* eating sequence and not with perfectionism.

To sum it up, as you eat *toward* your carbs, you will:

➤ Begin with low-carb protein and low-carb vegetables (from our low-carb lists).

➤ Next, move to higher-carb vegetables (vegetables *not* on our low-carb list) along with starchy foods (bread, rice, potatoes, and pasta, etc.).

➤ Finish off with sweets if they're part of your usual meal. (Fruit/fruit juice count as sweets.)

At each meal or snack, maintain the one-third rule of Day #3. Just remember to eat these foods in the order recommended: from low-carb to high-carb.* If you find that you are so satisfied that you simply don't want all the food you planned on eating, feel free not to eat it. It's up to you, but remember: if you cut down on the amount of food you eat at a meal, cut a bit off every type of food or, even better, eat less of the carbohydrate-rich food.

A Question Of Drink

Whether or not they contain carbohydrates, alcoholic beverages are metabolized along similar pathways. We consider them to be

---

*For a fun, new way to see how foods rank carb-wise, turn to page 152 for an easy, at-a-glance chart from our *Carbohydrate Addict's Carbohydrate Counter*.

Carbohydrate Act-Alikes.* In keeping with this Guideline, please hold off on—that is, delay consuming any—alcoholic beverages until after you have finished the low-carb protein and low-carb vegetable portion of your meal or snack. This request may seem unusual, but it can make a big difference in your cravings and weight loss. You can still enjoy your favorite wine or beer with dinner, just have it with your pasta, after you've finished your salad and chicken.

In the same way, sweetened soft drinks or beverages such as tea and coffee to which sugar or sugar substitute has been added are best consumed toward the latter part of a meal or snack, after you have eaten your low-carb protein, low-carb vegetables, and starchy foods. In the early part of your meal, it is best to drink a beverage that contains no sugar. Water, sparkling water, seltzer, unsweetened iced tea (with or without lemon), iced or hot coffee (with or without milk) fit the bill. Beverages containing sugar substitutes are best left to the latter part of the meal. Their sweet taste often fools the body into thinking it is getting sugar and into releasing insulin. The same goes for other food that includes these sweeteners.

The Pleasures Of Condiments

Condiments can add zip and pleasure to any meal, high-carb or low-carb. From plain old salt and pepper (exotic in their day) to spice blends that bear celebrity chefs' names, from chutneys and olives to a variety of salsas, condiments have become a mainstay of today's eating. In the past, the term "condiment" referred to an item added to food to enhance its flavor (herbs, spices, and the like). Today's more sophisticated and indulged diner has come to assume the right to a whole palette of goodies from around the world and refers to them, in the colloquial, as condiments.

---

*For more information on Carbohydrate Act-Alikes, including alcohol, sugar substitutes, and glutamates, see the "Five Vital Clues Low-Carb Diet Doctors Miss" chapter in this book.

Most of us have favorite foods that we enjoy at home or at our favorite restaurants—a special salsa with our chips, dill pickles at the deli, olives from our favorite Italian restaurant, the hot sauce we must have on our eggs. They are part of our private arsenal of pleasure, and most of us don't want anyone to ask us to give them up (and we won't!).

On the other hand, some condiments contain enough carbohydrates to turn a low-carb meal into a high-carb splurge. So before you pour on the ketchup or dig into the cranberry sauce, check to see if it should be considered a high-carb food. Our *Carbohydrate Addict's Carbohydrate Counter** can help you see in an instant the carbohydrate levels of a wide range of condiments, but feel free to choose any low-carb counter that you know you can rely on.

While following any of our 7-Day Jump-Start Guidelines, if a condiment is low-carb, you can continue to eat it as often as you like. If, on the other hand, it's high in carbohydrates, treat it as you would any high-carb food in this plan.

DAY #4 EXAMPLES

Old *Breakfast Using* *Prior Guidelines*	*New* *Day #4* *Breakfast*
A SMALL BAGEL WITH CREAM CHEESE 2 SCRAMBLED EGGS COFFEE WITH MILK (Eaten in any order as desired)	2 SCRAMBLED EGGS COFFEE WITH MILK *THEN* A SMALL BAGEL WITH CREAM CHEESE REMAINING COFFEE WITH MILK

---

*For a sample page of carb rankings from our *Carbohydrate Addict's Carbohydrate Counter* at-a-glance charts, see page 152 of this book.

Old *Lunch Using* *Prior Guidelines*	*New* *Day #4* *Lunch*
SMALL ROLL AND BUTTER LARGE SALAD WITH BUTTERMILK DRESSING (See Recipe Chapter) ½ ROTISSERIE CHICKEN SMALL COKE ½ LARGE CHOCOLATE CHIP COOKIE (Eaten in any order as desired)	LARGE SALAD WITH BUTTERMILK DRESSING (See Recipe Chapter) ½ ROTISSERIE CHICKEN *THEN* SMALL ROLL AND BUTTER *THEN* ½ LARGE CHOCOLATE CHIP COOKIE SMALL COKE
Old *Dinner Using* *Prior Guidelines*	*New* *Day #4* *Dinner*
CAESAR SALAD SHRIMP DIJON APPETIZER (See Recipe Chapter) SMALL GARLIC BREAD OR SIDE ORDER SPAGHETTI WITH SAUCE 3–4 MEATBALLS ASPARAGUS GLASS OF WINE PLATE OF FRESH FRUIT (Eaten in any order as desired)	CAESAR SALAD SHRIMP DIJON APPETIZER (See Recipe Chapter) 3–4 MEATBALLS ASPARAGUS *THEN* SMALL GARLIC BREAD OR SIDE ORDER SPAGHETTI WITH SAUCE GLASS OF WINE *THEN* PLATE OF FRESH FRUIT

(chart continues)

Old Late-Night Snack Using Prior Guidelines	*New Day #4 Late-Night Snack*
6–8 BUFFALO CHICKEN DRUMETTES	6–8 BUFFALO CHICKEN DRUMETTES
LARGE SIDE DISH OF CUCUMBER SLICES AND CELERY STICKS	LARGE SIDE DISH OF CUCUMBER SLICES AND CELERY STICKS
SMALL PORTION OF POTATO CHIPS	*THEN*
SMALL CHOCOLATE BAR	SMALL PORTION OF POTATO CHIPS
	THEN
(Eaten in any order as desired)	SMALL CHOCOLATE BAR

TROUBLE TAMER: DAY #4

The Guideline for Day #4 sounds easy enough, right? I mean, what does it take to eat your low-carb foods before you head for the high-carbs? You were almost doing that already, weren't you? So why, you wonder, didn't you follow the Guideline or why did you sorta-kinda follow it but not exactly?

Sometimes we are very funny creatures, we humans. If something is difficult, we tend to avoid it or, at least, put it off. On the other hand, when something seems easy, we often disregard its importance. After all, how much could "eating toward your carbs" really matter? The answer is . . . plenty!

Each Guideline serves a very important purpose, and all of them work together to get your body back into balance. So while it might not seem that difficult to eat toward your carbs, don't bypass this Guideline or assume that you can do it anytime you want. Once you've done it, we think you'll be surprised by how powerfully it affects the amount of food you desire and the reduction of cravings you experience.

Chapter 8

DAY #5: AS YOUR WEIGHT STARTS TO DROP

GUIDELINE: AT ALL *SNACKS*, EAT ONLY LOW-CARB FOODS.

Hold on and save all of your high-carb foods for meals only. Continue to follow all prior guidelines.

When you eat high-carb foods and your body releases insulin, your cells get ready to receive nourishment in the form of blood sugar. Put in basic terms, this energy moves in one direction, from the bloodstream into the cells of the muscles and organs. Whatever blood sugar remains (that is, whatever is not used by these cells) is then turned into blood fat and continues to move into other cells—this time, into fat cells.

So when your insulin levels are high, you are in a Saving Mode, moving energy in. The more often you eat high-carb foods, the more often you release insulin, and the longer you remain in a Saving Mode.

In order to lose weight, you have to get your body *out* of its Saving Mode and into a Spending Mode. This Guideline is designed to help you remain longer in a Spending (fat-burning, weight-loss) Mode. As the pounds continue to drop, you want to stay in the Spending Mode for as long as possible, while getting the nutrition you need to stay healthy and the pleasure you need to stay motivated.

Fortunately, that's not difficult. When you have *not* eaten high-carb foods for a while, your insulin levels drop. No longer flooded with insulin and blood sugar, your muscles and organs begin to run out of energy. Your body begins to turn the energy in your fat cells back into blood sugar and use it to fuel cells in the muscles and organs.

> Whether or not you lose weight or gain
> weight is determined not only by the
> *amount* of high-carb food you eat,
> but also by *how often* you eat it!

The longer insulin levels remain low (because you haven't eaten high-carb foods for a while), the more time your body has to release fat from the fat cells and burn it up. Each pound you lose is proof positive that your body has remained long enough in a Spending Mode to burn up some of its fat stores. In addition, and fortunately for us, nature has built a sort of "safety switch" into the system to allow us a little leeway.

In the last decade, scientists studying the way we store and burn fat have made a discovery that is extraordinarily important to any low-carb dieter. They have realized that whether you lose weight, stay at the same weight, or gain weight is determined not only by the *amount* of high-carb food you eat, but also by *how often* you eat it!

> Many low-carb diet doctors seem unaware
> that *how often* you eat carbohydrates is as
> important as *how much* of them you eat.

We call this phenomenon the Frequency Factor and although we, as well of other scientists, are very excited about the power of the Frequency Factor to influence weight gain or loss, as well as carbohydrate cravings, many low-carb diet doctors seem to be unaware of it.*

Day #5's Guideline uses the Frequency Factor to help you lose weight. You will be asked to *decrease* the number of times each day you eat high-carb foods so that you can keep your body in a Spending Mode for longer periods of time. Longer periods of spending mean greater weight loss and fewer cravings. (Your body doesn't need you to take in food while it's busy spending the energy you have already stored.) You will still be able to eat low-carb foods as before. We merely ask that you hold on and eat the high-carb foods less often.

We're amazed that the Frequency Factor is so rarely discussed. While everyone concentrates on how *much* carbohydrate they consume, most people are never told that *how often* they eat high-carb foods may be just as important (or more!).

If, for instance, you were to eat six cookies at a single sitting, the high-carb content of the cookies would be likely to raise your insulin levels, and put you into a Saving Mode, just once. On the other hand, if you were to divide those cookies into three snacks of two cookies each during the day, you would probably raise your insulin levels, and go into a Saving Mode, *three times!* To make matters worse, the shorter the time between snacks, the greater your insulin levels would rise each time. So by the third snack, you'd be experiencing an insulin surge with added punch and a longer-than-ever Saving Mode. You could probably expect your body to take quite a while to get back to a Spending Mode.

---

*You'll find more information on the Frequency Factor, and how it can allow you to enjoy carbs once a day and still lose weight, in the chapter "Five Vital Clues Low-Carb Diet Doctors Miss."

> Three alcoholic drinks consumed in a half hour will affect you differently than the same number consumed over several hours.
>
> The same is true for starches and sweets (though in a surprisingly different way).

Here's a real-life example that might make the Frequency Factor more understandable. You've probably noticed that timing has a big effect on the way the body handles alcohol consumption. Three drinks consumed very quickly can have a powerful effect on a person—they'll probably make the person intoxicated—whereas the same three drinks consumed over several hours, especially if they're taken with food, are less apt to make the person drunk. The same amount of alcohol, but radically different effects.

In the same way, the period of time in which you consume high-carb food can affect how your body metabolizes it. Your body is better able to handle the onslaught of high carbs at one sitting than if you were to nibble on them all day.

Some scientists have speculated that the reason our bodies can handle a single onslaught of high-carb foods goes back to the era of the caveman. For most of the time, the caveman's body was in a Spending Mode. His food was energy poor. He subsisted on the flesh of animals that had eaten only grasses, and therefore was lean and muscular. He supplemented his carnivorous feedings with a variety of energy-poor stems and leaves (those he knew he could eat without poisoning himself). Generally, his body immediately burned any food he found in order to fuel itself so that it could go out and find yet more food.

The discovery of a stash of high-carb food was very rare, most likely appearing in the form of fruit only a few weeks out of the year. If a great find of fruit was discovered, the caveman's body was able to move from the Spending Mode into a Saving Mode, stocking the fruit sugar away for future use. In order to store food energy, the caveman's body released insulin that, as you know, set the whole Saving process into action. In addition, however, the insulin surge brought about other reactions designed to prompt the caveman to get the most out of his high-carb find.

When high-carb foods were found in abundance and eaten for prolonged periods, or if they were eaten frequently throughout the day, great surges of insulin would signal the body to move into the Saving Mode. Cravings would increase, energy levels would drop, and our caveman would be content to stay where he was, eat to his heart's content, fall into a sugar-induced stupor, and sleep it off while his body went to work, filling up his fat cells. When he awakened, he would find himself irresistibly drawn to the fruit once again, and the entire process would begin again, to be repeated until the source of the fruit had been consumed completely.

In the event that only a small amount of high-carb food was available, however, and our caveman needed to remain capable of finding or hunting down other sources of food, his body developed the ability to judge the situation and make changes accordingly. If only a small amount of high-carb food was consumed, assuming that the reduced amount was all that was available, the body remained in a Spending Mode. Less insulin was released and with it, fewer cravings for high-carb foods. Less of a sense of tiredness followed the consumption of smaller amounts of fruit. If there was not enough fruit at hand to stock up the caveman's fat cells, it would have been counterproductive to send messages that encouraged him to sleep.

As a final backup, given the possibility that sources of high-carb food might be scattered in small amounts across a limited area, the caveman developed a system that reacted to the repeated intake of food like fruit, even in small amounts, in the same way it reacted to an abundance discovered in a single setting. So if he were to eat a food such as fruit over and over, even in limited quantities, our caveman's body released repeated surges of insulin, moving him into the Saving Mode.

This basic Saving and Spending system, and the high-carbs that trigger the insulin surges that set it in motion, plays an important role in what you experience every day; every time you see, smell, or think about high-carb foods and find the experience enjoyable, every time a mint or piece of gum crosses your lips and tastes pleasant, you are experiencing an insulin surge. Of most importance to you, however, may be the fact that when you give up your favorite high-carb foods instead of simply using your body's own ability to *disregard* the once-in-a-while intake of high-carb foods, you are needlessly sacrificing your pleasure. The essential word here is *infrequent.* On an *infrequent* basis your body will accommodate a moderate intake of high-carb food.

How infrequent? In other words, how often can you eat high-carb food without producing great surges of insulin that put it into a long-term Saving Mode?

Scientists have discovered that the average person can eat high-carb food once a day and still remain able to burn energy by staying in a Spending Mode. We have also confirmed that three criteria must be met: (1) the high-carbohydrate content of the meal must be moderate in size; (2) a balance of low-carb protein and, ideally, low-carb high-fiber vegetables and/or salad must be present; and (3) the meal must be consumed within a limited period of time, preferably within one hour.*

The purpose of Day #5's Guideline and the two remaining Guidelines that follow is simply to allow you to remain in the Spending Mode longer, burning up the energy you take in as well as the energy stored in your fat cells, and to decrease your cravings so that you desire fewer high-carb foods. Decreasing the *frequency*—that is, the number of times each day—with which you eat high-carb foods is essential to lowering cravings and raising weight loss.

You will still get to enjoy your favorite high-carb foods— bread, pasta, potatoes, cake, donuts, ice cream, fruit, even

---

*This final criteria, the one-hour time limit on the intake of high-carb foods, is an important area we address in detail in our Carbohydrate Addict's LifeSpan Program. If you are considering moving to that eating plan upon completing your 7-Day Jump-Start Plan, or if your meals extend to more than an hour, please consult *The Carbohydrate Addict's LifeSpan Program.*

candy—but along with the previous Guidelines that helped you to balance them with low-carb protein and fiber, you will be asked to save them for fewer meals.

So if you've ever said, "I could stay on a diet, really stick with it, if I could just have the food I love *sometimes!*" here's your chance.

For Day #5, you are asked to save all high-carb foods for meals only. That means, no high-carbs during snacks.

If you're not sure what constitutes a meal versus a snack, consider your three largest intakes of food to be meals. Anything else is a snack, and during these snacks, hold on and do not have any high-carb foods. As you follow this Guideline, you will have high-carb food no more than three times a day (while continuing to follow all prior Guidelines) and you'll begin to move your body from a Saving Mode into a Spending Mode.

Displacing And Replacing Carbs

A hold-on, like Day #5's Guideline, which asks you to save your high-carb foods for another time, is *not* asking you to give up a full and satisfying snack or meal. When you remove high-carb foods from a snack or meal, you are welcome to replace them with additional low-carb proteins and low-carb vegetables and/or salad in keeping with previous Guidelines.

Beverages

Most low-carb weight-loss programs give you free rein to consume all the sugar substitute you wish at any meal or snack, or in between. We have found that consuming sugar substitutes can lead to cravings for high-carb foods and slow your weight loss.* We recommend that at all low-carb meals and snacks (and in between) you consume food or drink that is free of sugar

---

*You'll find more information on all of the Carbohydrate Act-Alikes, including sugar substitutes, in Chapter 12, "Five Vital Clues Low-Carb Diet Doctors Miss."

substitutes of any kind in order to get the full craving-reducing and weight-loss benefits.

When You're In The Lead

What should you do if you are already eating high-carb foods only three times a day (or fewer) or if you are eating nothing but three meals a day (or fewer)? In that case, this Guideline requires no change. First, be certain that you are not, in fact, eating high-carb foods at more than three meals a day (including any snacks). If this is so, you can either move to Day #6 or consider Day #5 to be one in which you need to change nothing and just continue with the Guidelines you have already been following. Don't put pressure on yourself in either direction. Follow your preference. This is your life and your success.

DAY #5 EXAMPLES

Old Breakfast *Using Prior Guidelines*	*New* *Day #5 Breakfast*
2 SCRAMBLED EGGS	2 SCRAMBLED EGGS
COFFEE WITH MILK	COFFEE WITH MILK
THEN	*THEN*
A SMALL BAGEL WITH CREAM CHEESE	A SMALL BAGEL WITH CREAM CHEESE
REMAINING COFFEE WITH MILK	REMAINING COFFEE WITH MILK
	(No change needed)

Old Lunch *Using Prior Guidelines*	*New* *Day #5 Lunch*
LARGE SALAD WITH BUTTERMILK DRESSING (See Recipe Chapter)	LARGE SALAD WITH BUTTERMILK DRESSING (See Recipe Chapter)
½ ROTISSERIE CHICKEN	½ ROTISSERIE CHICKEN
THEN	*THEN*
SMALL ROLL AND BUTTER	SMALL ROLL AND BUTTER
THEN	*THEN*
½ LARGE CHOCOLATE CHIP COOKIE	½ LARGE CHOCOLATE CHIP COOKIE
SMALL COKE	SMALL COKE
	(No change needed)
Old Dinner *Using Prior Guidelines*	*New* *Day #5 Dinner*
CAESAR SALAD	CAESAR SALAD
SHRIMP DIJON APPETIZER (See Recipe Chapter)	SHRIMP DIJON APPETIZER (See Recipe Chapter)
3–4 MEATBALLS	3–4 MEATBALLS
ASPARAGUS	ASPARAGUS
THEN	*THEN*
SMALL GARLIC BREAD OR SIDE ORDER SPAGHETTI WITH SAUCE	SMALL GARLIC BREAD OR SIDE ORDER SPAGHETTI WITH SAUCE
GLASS OF WINE	GLASS OF WINE
THEN	*THEN*
PLATE OF FRESH FRUIT	PLATE OF FRESH FRUIT
	(No change needed)

(chart continues)

Old Late-Night Snack Using Prior Guidelines	*New Day #5 Late-Night Snack*
6–8 BUFFALO CHICKEN DRUMETTES	6–8 BUFFALO CHICKEN DRUMETTES
LARGE SIDE DISH OF CUCUMBER SLICES AND CELERY STICKS	LARGE SIDE DISH OF CUCUMBER SLICES AND CELERY STICKS
THEN	WEDGE OF NEW ORLEANS CRUSTLESS QUICHE* (See Recipe Chapter)
SMALL PORTION OF POTATO CHIPS	
THEN	
SMALL CHOCOLATE BAR	

TROUBLE TAMER: DAY #5

Many people actually welcome this Guideline at first, saying they are happy to be in the swing of things, obviously moving toward a low-carb eating plan. Others encounter resistance they didn't expect. If you had difficulty giving up high-carb foods at all snacks in Day #5, please be certain you have been following all of the previous Guidelines. They have been designed to get your body ready to let go of high-carb foods and, if you've been fudging on any of them (no pun intended), your body may be in a state of insulin imbalance, making it harder for you to resist high-carb foods.

So first reread the previous Guidelines. If, indeed, you need to brush up on them, take a day or two to be certain you're following them correctly. If, on the other hand, you've been following the Guidelines to a "T," make sure that you've been allowing enough time to prepare the food you need (when you need it) rather than "making do" with whatever low-carb foods you find handy.

Day #5 is an important transition Guideline, so give yourself any extra time you may need to get it right before moving on.

---

*Today's Guideline requires you to hold off on high-carb foods during all snacks. If desired, low-carb food may be added in their place.

DAY #6:
SUCCESS IN SIGHT

GUIDELINE: AT ALL SNACKS *AND* AT ONE MEAL EAT ONLY LOW-CARB FOODS.

Hold on and have all of your high-carb foods at no more than two meals daily. Continue to follow all prior guidelines.

For Day #6, you are asked to hold on and include all high-carb foods in no more than two meals in a day. That means only low-carb proteins, vegetables, and/or salads during snacks and during one of your meals.

Choose any two meals today as your Reward Meals, that is, meals in which high-carb foods are included in balance with low-carb foods (as described in the Guideline for Day #3). During Reward Meals, eat toward your carbs (as described in the Guideline for Day #4). We encourage you to decide at the start of the day which of your meals will be your Reward Meals.

If, for instance, you make a commitment to have your Reward Meals at breakfast and dinner (and plan on having only low-carb foods at lunch and at any snacks), try to avoid spontaneously deciding at lunch to make that your Reward Meal in place of a Reward Meal dinner.

Should something unexpected arise—an unanticipated lunch out, for instance—you are still free to change your Reward Meal to lunch, but it's best to decide as far ahead of time as possible, then make plans for ensuring that your dinner will remain free of high-carbs. For each span of time you hold on and eat only low-carb foods, you are telling your body it needs less time Saving and more time Spending the energy it has stored away in your fat cells.

Been There, Doing That, And Loving It

If you are already eating high-carb foods only twice a day (or less), or if you generally eat only two meals a day (or fewer), you are already meeting this Guideline. Chances are you are beginning to experience freedom from recurring and intense cravings and are moving toward your weight-loss goal. Since you are already meeting Day #6's Guideline, you can either move to Day #7 now or you can consider Day #6 to be a day in which you need to change nothing while continuing to follow all prior Guidelines.

A Plan With A Purpose

The purpose of the Guidelines for Day #6 and Day #7 is to help you remain even longer in the Spending Mode, to better burn the energy stored in your fat cells, and by helping to balance your insulin levels, to decrease your cravings so that staying on your eating plan becomes easier and easier.

For Day #6, you are asked to hold on and save all high-carb foods for two meals only. Remember that when you remove high-carb foods from a meal, you are welcome to replace them with additional low-carb proteins and low-carb vegetables and/or salad in keeping with previous Guidelines.

DAY #6 EXAMPLES

Old Breakfast *Using Prior Guidelines*	*New* *Day #6 Breakfast*
2 SCRAMBLED EGGS COFFEE WITH MILK *THEN* A SMALL BAGEL WITH CREAM CHEESE REMAINING COFFEE WITH MILK	2 SCRAMBLED EGGS COFFEE WITH MILK *THEN* A SMALL BAGEL WITH CREAM CHEESE REMAINING COFFEE WITH MILK (One of today's two Reward Meals. No change needed)
Old Lunch *Using Prior Guidelines*	*New* *Day #6 Lunch*
LARGE SALAD WITH BUTTERMILK DRESSING (See Recipe Chapter) ½ ROTISSERIE CHICKEN *THEN* SMALL ROLL AND BUTTER *THEN* ½ LARGE CHOCOLATE CHIP COOKIE SMALL COKE	LOW-CARB ITALIAN BREAD* (See Recipe Chapter) LARGE SALAD WITH BUTTERMILK DRESSING (See Recipe Chapter) ½ ROTISSERIE CHICKEN TUNA-STUFFED MUSHROOMS (See Recipe Chapter)

(chart continues)

*Today's Guideline requires you to hold off on high-carbs at one additional meal. We've chosen lunch as that meal and have removed all high-carb food from it, while adding low-carb food. At breakfast and dinner (Reward Meals) we are continuing to include high-carb foods.

Old Dinner *Using Prior Guidelines*	*New* *Day #6 Dinner*
CAESAR SALAD	CAESAR SALAD
SHRIMP DIJON APPETIZER (See Recipe Chapter)	SHRIMP DIJON APPETIZER (See Recipe Chapter)
3–4 MEATBALLS	3–4 MEATBALLS
ASPARAGUS	ASPARAGUS
THEN	*THEN*
SMALL GARLIC BREAD OR SIDE ORDER OF SPAGHETTI WITH SAUCE	SMALL GARLIC BREAD OR SIDE ORDER OF SPAGHETTI WITH SAUCE
GLASS OF WINE	GLASS OF WINE
THEN	*THEN*
PLATE OF FRESH FRUIT	PLATE OF FRESH FRUIT
	(No change needed)
Old Late-Night Snack *Using Prior Guidelines*	*New Day #6* *Late-Night Snack*
6–8 BUFFALO CHICKEN DRUMETTES	6–8 BUFFALO CHICKEN DRUMETTES
LARGE SIDE DISH OF CUCUMBER SLICES AND CELERY STICKS	LARGE SIDE DISH OF CUCUMBER SLICES AND CELERY STICKS
WEDGE OF NEW ORLEANS CRUSTLESS QUICHE (See Recipe Chapter)	WEDGE OF NEW ORLEANS CRUSTLESS QUICHE (See Recipe Chapter)
	(No change needed)

The Lure Of Routine: Avoid It!

As you begin to eat snacks and then meals that contain only low-carb food, be certain to put extra effort into making these dishes taste really special. Although you may think you are just as happy having the same piece of steak and steamed vegetables or plain salad day after day, you will get tired of them.

> Like everyone else, low-carb
> dieters need exciting food.

People fall off their low-carb programs not from hunger, but from a need for excitement. Instead of realizing that you're getting tired of the same old uninteresting regime, you may tell yourself that your way of eating is "good enough," or even worse, that it's "easy." We have found that low-carb weight-loss success is not only about staying on track today; it's about making your program so enjoyable that you'll stay on track tomorrow.

We have found that nine out of ten low-carb dieters eat the same basic meal of plain protein and veggies for lunch and dinner (and snacks and breakfast too). Although low-carb cookbooks abound and low-carb dieters buy them "for ideas," few actually try the recipes and incorporate them into their diets.

> If you don't make your low-carb food exciting,
> you'll soon be on the prowl for something
> more interesting—and that's sure to be
> a high-carb food.

Imagine going to a restaurant that only served plain meat and vegetables at every meal, every day. Boring! We can't tell you how important it is to vary your low-carb dishes and to make them fun.

If you don't think low-carb proteins, vegetables, and salads can be interesting, you need to come to our house for dinner. A typical meal for us starts off with a Shrimp Picatta appetizer, followed by a Chicken Caesar Salad. The main course might include both a steak and green pepper stir-fry (left over from yesterday) and a bubbling cheese-topped Chicken Parmesan. Green beans with Richard's favorite spicy sauce round out the meal, although we always include a side plate of raw vegetables (to satisfy the need to crunch!) and our favorite low-carb dipping sauce.

TROUBLE TAMER: DAY #6

Day #6's Guideline isn't difficult to understand. It is a direct extension of Day #5's. Day #6 requires you to save your high-carb food and enjoy it at two Reward Meals only.

Some people welcome this step. It means they are that much closer to their weight-loss goal, and as they proceed, their cravings continue to disappear. They may also enjoy their newfound sense of control and the emerging belief that what they formerly considered to be a lack of willpower was, indeed, a physical imbalance.

Others, however, may need some time to adjust. If you had difficulty fully meeting Day #6's Guideline, allow yourself the freedom to experiment with your choice of time, type of food, and setting in which to eat your low-carb meal.

For one person, a low-carb breakfast might be simple. Celery stuffed with cream cheese and a quick cup of coffee might easily do the trick. For another, however, giving up a full breakfast complete with toast and cereal might prove, at this time, too much of a sacrifice. In the former scenario, breakfast is an excellent choice for a low-carb meal to meet today's Guideline. In the latter scenario, however, lunch—which often consists of meat, salad, and bread—might be a better starting place, since a second vegetable could be substituted for the bread.

So give yourself some latitude. Take a day or two if you need it to make some good choices before you move on to your next (and last) Guideline.

Chapter 10

DAY #7: HAVING YOUR CAKE AND LOSING WEIGHT TOO

First, a note: After you integrate this final Guideline into your eating and you have completed Day #7, you will be moving into the "Continuing Success" portion of this plan.

In "Continuing Success" we will help you keep moving toward your eating and weight-loss goals, giving you the tips, tactics, and troubleshooting strategies you will need to continue your success.

GUIDELINE: AT TWO MEALS *AND* AT ALL SNACKS
EAT ONLY LOW-CARB FOODS.

> Hold on and have all of your high-carb foods at
> only one meal each day (your Reward Meal).
> Continue to follow all prior guidelines.

Day #7's Guideline asks that you hold on and include all high-carb foods in one meal only. That means eat only low-carbohydrate proteins, vegetables, and/or salads during snacks and at all meals with the exception of the one meal you choose as your Reward Meal.

You may choose any meal to be your Reward Meal—dinner, for example, after deciding that you'd love that piece of lemon meringue pie you noticed in the refrigerator. Or perhaps you're in the mood for Italian food and choose lunch with a friend at your favorite restaurant as your Reward Meal. Many people enjoy a Reward Breakfast, especially if it's a day when they don't have to work and can take the time to make it special and un-rushed. Whatever meal you choose as your Reward Meal is up to you. Just make certain to balance your high-carbohydrate foods with low-carbohydrate proteins, vegetables, and/or salads and to always eat toward your carbs.

As you know from Day #6, it is always best to decide in advance which of your meals will be your Reward Meal and plan for it to be a special treat. Although temptation may strike at other times, we think you'll find it far easier to resist when you know that you can have the food you love at your Reward Meal. Again, it's better not to spontaneously make a low-carb meal into a Reward Meal simply because there is a high-carb food you suddenly want to eat. On the other hand, if you are caught unaware, and simply cannot resist having a high-carbohydrate food at a meal that was supposed to be all low-carbohydrate, consider that meal to be your Reward Meal and change your intended Reward Meal into a low-carbohydrate meal instead. Remember that for each span of time you hold on and eat only low-carb foods, your body will spend less time Saving and more time Spending the energy stored in your fat cells.

> A snack of just potato chips or candy (or both)
> does not a balanced Reward Meal make.

No Push To Rush

If, before you arrive at Day #7, you have been having your carbohydrate-rich foods only once a day, you *may* find that the Guideline for Day #7 requires no change. Before you make that determination, however, check to see that the one time at which you eat high-carb foods each day takes the form of a balanced meal in which you eat toward your high-carb foods. A snack of just potato chips or candy (or both) does not a balanced Reward Meal make. If you are *indulging* in a spontaneous (or even a planned) high-carb treat each day and that treat is not balanced with low-carb foods that you eat first, you are not yet fulfilling Day #7's Guideline. In that case, plan to have your treat at the end of a balanced meal and make the entire experience a reward.

On the other hand, if this Guideline offers no change from your usual routine, once again you have two choices. You can turn to the "Continuing Success" chapter of this book and begin to make the transition (at your own pace) to the eating plan you would like to continue (including one that gives you the option of a daily Reward Meal), or you can remain at this step (in which a daily Reward Meal is expected). As always, you should be guided by your own preferences and not the expectations of others.

Remember that when you remove high-carb food from a meal, you are welcome to replace it with additional low-carb proteins and low-carb vegetables and/or salad, in keeping with previous Guidelines.

A Seamless Transition

At this point, your insulin and blood sugar levels should be in far greater balance than they were on Day #1. You'll most likely be experiencing far fewer cravings and your body will have begun to burn up the energy you've stored in your fat cells.

> In most cases, it is something in the food
> you are eating that has driven you to go
> off your diet rather than some lack
> of willpower on your part.

If you are still having intense or recurring cravings, either on a regular basis or on occasion, make certain to read Chapter 13, "Hidden Carbs . . . Waiting to Pounce," and Chapter 15, "Trouble-Shooting." In most cases, it is something in the food you are eating that has driven you to go off your diet rather than some lack of willpower on your part. Before blaming yourself, look first for the outside trigger that may be setting off your insulin surges.

If you're convinced that you're not losing weight, be aware that daily fluctuations in weight can mask real weight loss. Many people make the mistake of reacting to daily changes in weight as if they were permanent, when we all know we can gain or lose a couple of pounds depending on a wide variety of factors, including how salty a meal was. In order to stay on track, you need an accurate way of judging your weight loss; see Chapter 15 for a full explanation.

You can move into the "Continuing Success" chapter as soon as you have completed Day #7 of this plan, where, if you like, you can continue to enjoy the benefits of eating according to Day #7's Guidelines.

It is important, however, not to assume that Day #7 completes your plan. If you want to continue to enjoy a daily Reward Meal and lose weight on a program you can stick with for life, there is a great deal more you need to know. On the other hand, if you want to return to your previous low-carb program, you'll need some guidance. In either case, as soon as you've completed this Guideline, it's time to move onto your "Continuing Success" (the experience as well as the next chapter.) We'll see you there!

DAY #7 EXAMPLES

Old Breakfast *Using Prior Guidelines*	*New* *Day #7 Breakfast*
2 SCRAMBLED EGGS	2 SCRAMBLED EGGS
COFFEE WITH MILK	COFFEE WITH MILK
THEN	INSTANT BREAKFAST SAUSAGE*
A SMALL BAGEL WITH CREAM CHEESE	(See Recipe Chapter)
REMAINING COFFEE WITH MILK	

---

*Today's Guideline requires you to hold off on high-carbs at all meals and snacks except one meal. We've chosen breakfast as our new low-carb meal and have removed all high-carb foods from this meal while adding low-carb foods as desired. We continue with lunch as a low-carb meal. At dinner (our Reward Meal), we are continuing to include high-carb foods.

Old Lunch *Using Prior Guidelines*	*New* *Day #7 Lunch*
LOW-CARB ITALIAN BREAD (See Recipe Chapter) LARGE SALAD WITH BUTTERMILK DRESSING (See Recipe Chapter) ½ ROTISSERIE CHICKEN TUNA-STUFFED MUSHROOMS (See Recipe Chapter)	LOW-CARB ITALIAN BREAD (See Recipe Chapter) LARGE SALAD WITH BUTTERMILK DRESSING (See Recipe Chapter) ½ ROTISSERIE CHICKEN TUNA-STUFFED MUSHROOMS (See Recipe Chapter) (No change needed)
Old Dinner *Using Prior Guidelines*	*New* *Day #7 Dinner*
CAESAR SALAD SHRIMP DIJON APPETIZER (See Recipe Chapter) 3–4 MEATBALLS ASPARAGUS *THEN* SMALL GARLIC BREAD OR SIDE ORDER SPAGHETTI WITH SAUCE GLASS OF WINE *THEN* PLATE OF FRESH FRUIT	CAESAR SALAD SHRIMP DIJON APPETIZER (See Recipe Chapter) 3–4 MEATBALLS ASPARAGUS *THEN* SMALL GARLIC BREAD OR SIDE ORDER SPAGHETTI WITH SAUCE GLASS OF WINE *THEN* PLATE OF FRESH FRUIT (Reward Meal; no change needed)

(chart continues)

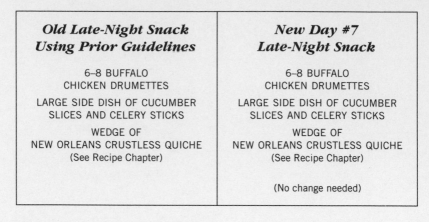

Old Late-Night Snack Using Prior Guidelines	*New Day #7 Late-Night Snack*
6–8 BUFFALO CHICKEN DRUMETTES	6–8 BUFFALO CHICKEN DRUMETTES
LARGE SIDE DISH OF CUCUMBER SLICES AND CELERY STICKS	LARGE SIDE DISH OF CUCUMBER SLICES AND CELERY STICKS
WEDGE OF NEW ORLEANS CRUSTLESS QUICHE (See Recipe Chapter)	WEDGE OF NEW ORLEANS CRUSTLESS QUICHE (See Recipe Chapter)
	(No change needed)

TROUBLE TAMER: DAY #7

While the Guidelines for Day #6 and Day #7 are almost the same, the experience of delaying high-carbs in two of three meals, rather than just one, can feel quite different. Some people jump into the last of the Guidelines feet first. Their insulin in balance and cravings gone, they are ready to forge ahead.

Others find it a big change, and are often unsure as to which of the two remaining meals to make low-carb. If that is your concern, we recommend that you experiment. Give yourself a few days to try out different combinations of low-carb versus high-carb timings. On workdays, for instance, you may find that a quick low-carb breakfast and a simple low-carb lunch fit perfectly into your lifestyle and satisfy you as long as you know your Reward Dinner is waiting for you as soon as you get home in the evening. Weekends away from work, however, may rekindle your love of a full and leisurely high-carb breakfast, while you don't consider it a sacrifice to stick to steak, chicken, or fish and appropriate low-carb vegetables and salads at your low-carb lunch and dinner.

If you didn't follow today's Guideline as you think you should have, or if you just need a day or two to feel comfortable and secure at this point in the Plan, then take the time to do it right before you move on to the next chapter and to your Continuing Success.

Chapter 11

CONTINUING SUCCESS

Well, you've made it! Seven days (more or less), seven steps (more or less), and you've taken your body from a state of chaos (or, at least, confusion) into a state in which it can work toward getting you to a normal, healthy weight.

While you've been working on balancing your body, your mind has not been far behind. Each Guideline has helped control your body's drive for high-carb foods while your mind was gaining self-confidence in your ability to stay on an eating program.

Freedom from recurring and intense cravings and a renewed sense of self-control are just a few of the many wonderful experiences you should have enjoyed as you moved from Day #1 through Day #7 of the 7-Day Jump-Start Plan. If, for any reason, you did *not* or are *not* experiencing a definite and significant decrease in your cravings and a far greater feeling of self-control over food, there may be something (or many things) that you are eating that is (are) triggering your impulse to eat high-carbohydrate foods.

> Whenever you experience intense cravings, chances are something you ate is throwing your insulin levels out of balance.

In that case, it is essential that you ferret out those items in your meals or snacks that are causing your body to crave foods (in particular, high-carbs). Unless you put in the effort needed to determine the culprits that are pushing you to eat (and gain weight easily), you are likely to, once again, throw up your hands and assume that like all the programs that have failed you before, this plan has not brought you struggle-free weight loss. We can't find the culprits for you. You have to do it, once and for all, or you may never break free of the belief that it is you or your program that has failed rather than something you are eating.

If you are troubled by recurring cravings and/or weight gain, we encourage you to take the time and, using the help we offer in our books, methodically examine the food you're eating. In an overwhelmingly great percentage of cases, our readers are able to identify most (if not all) of the trigger foods (or the unnecessary ingredients that have been added to them) that are throwing their bodies out of balance. Generally, these same readers are able to substitute similar foods, or those that are prepared without triggering additives or ingredients, so that they can move on to a craving-free weight loss.

Other readers, however, remain stalwart, refusing to believe that cravings can be caused by anything except their own lack of self-control. Try as we might to convince them otherwise, so intent on blaming themselves, so wedded to the blame-the-victim mentality that is rampant these days, that they would rather throw away their chance at true freedom than change their long-held belief in their own worthlessness.

Imagine for a moment that every time you ate strawberries, you broke out in a rash. The more often you ate the strawberries, the worse the rash became. Imagine, too, that it got to a point that if you ate even a small amount of strawberries, you'd be covered—from head to toe—in a rash. It seems obvious that, looking at this chain of events, you would assume that you had a "sensitivity" or allergy to strawberries. You would not blame yourself for breaking out in a rash, think of the rash or your desire to scratch it as a sign of moral weakness, or feel ashamed of the fact that, although others could eat strawberries without repercussions, you simply could not.

If you are carbohydrate sensitive,
the hidden carbohydrates or the additives
in your food could be pushing you
to eat—against your will.

We wonder, then, why it is so difficult to believe that for those who are carbohydrate sensitive, eating certain foods (in particular, those that are high in carbohydrates), either in great amounts or too frequently, can cause them to "break out" in carbohydrate cravings and weight gain. Although the experience of having a far more intense and compelling need for carbohydrates may have led the former surgeon general of the United States to use the term "carbohydrate sensitive" to describe such people, those who have this imbalance often can't admit to themselves that they might not be at fault.

Ironically, no matter how logical the strawberry analogy is, we often see a mixed reaction on the face of the person we're addressing with it.

On one hand, people know that what we are saying is true. "I know that I'm different," they tell us. "My husband eats a couple pieces of candy and he's finished. I eat the same couple of pieces and I just can't stop."

Yet these same people, who know they react to food differently than family and friends, on finding themselves experiencing intense and compelling cravings, do not look to see which foods might have "set them off" in the direction of the high-carb hunt. Instead, they revert to old self-blame scripts that have never prompted them to discover the *cause* of their cravings.

So we request the following of you. If, after completing the 7-Day Jump-Start Plan, you still have intense or recurring cravings on a regular basis, or if—at any time in the future—you should suddenly find yourself unable to control your eating (or that it takes great effort to do so), take the time to find the *cause* of your cravings. Within the many chapters in this book, you will discover information, tips, and revelations that have been hard won by ourselves and others. Use them to free yourself not only from your cravings but from the cycle of self-blame as well.

You may find that a certain food eaten one time does not lead to cravings, but when the same food is eaten on more than one occasion, you may experience an irresistible urge to eat every high-carb in sight. That's not as unusual as it sounds.

Going back to the strawberry analogy, imagine that eating strawberries on a rare occasion does not make you break out in a rash, but that eating them at breakfast, lunch, and dinner covers you with hives from head to toe. You'd be likely to conclude that, while you can tolerate them under certain circumstances, you are, indeed, still sensitive to the strawberries. Furthermore, although other people can eat them as often as they like without negative repercussions, your body simply is not built that way.

In the same way, some people are more sensitive than others to high-carb food. For them, starches, snack foods, and sweets (and for some, in particular, fruit and fruit juice), can upset their body's balance. They can eat these foods once a day without a strong physical reaction, but not more often.

It is estimated that four out of five people who struggle with their weight have a sensitivity to carbohydrates. If, indeed, you find yourself craving carbohydrates, although you are eating high-carb foods only once a day in a balanced meal, then the reason for your cravings is almost certainly one of two things: either you are eating carbohydrates more often than once a day without knowing it, or other ingredients in your foods are triggering your carbohydrate sensitivity.

You will find important information in Chapter 13, "Hidden Carbs . . . Waiting to Pounce." This chapter contains vital facts about ingredients in your food that you may assume are harmless but which may be keeping you from achieving success.

So the next time you feel cravings that make you want to reach for the carbs, reach for this book instead. Instead of blaming yourself, become your own Sherlock Holmes; discover the culprits that have been robbing you of your willpower, your happiness, and your weight loss all these years. We put in the time and energy to dig out the saboteurs in our own food, and it was more than worth the effort. It made our continuing success that much easier, and we want the same for you.

The Paths Before You

"What do I do now?" is a welcome question we often hear. It's the best of all questions because it implies you have a choice (one of the world's most blessed situations!).

First, let's get a little perspective. When you started this plan, you sought help to regain control of your eating and, in doing so, jump-start your weight loss.

Now that you've incorporated all of the Guidelines of the 7-Day Jump-Start Plan, it's essential that you take some time to savor that achievement. For some reason, when we do something well, we tend to take it for granted. Don't you do that!

"Okay, I did it," you say. "So what's next?"

The answer is to look at what you did right and learn from it. That's correct: what you did right.

Did you take more time than usual in caring of yourself? Did you put your needs before those of other people? Did you start your plan when you were off work or when you otherwise had extra time to prepare your meals? Did you treat yourself with extra money or extra effort in order to give yourself the food you most enjoy?

Keep in mind whatever steps you took to get yourself successfully to this point, and use them again for your continued success.

Your Just Rewards

Before you decide how you would like to continue, we urge you to listen not only to logic but to your heart as well. That's one of the rewards—the rights—that you've earned. You've proven that with the correct help, you can do what you always knew you could do.

While you might conclude that it would be "easier" or "more

logical" to follow one low-carb program rather than another, if your heart says you really don't want to follow it, in the end that voice will likely cast the final vote. No matter how easy a plan is, if it isn't one you can live with—or that you *want* to live with—you're not going to stay with it.

Sometimes it's hard to know what we want. We're so busy telling ourselves why we *can't* have what we want that we fail to recognize when we *can* have it. For a moment, imagine all of the low-carb diets you've ever been on and allow yourself to experience how you feel about returning to each one of them. Try not to talk yourself out of the feelings, just make note of them.

Now, picture what you want in a low-carb diet. Not just the results but in the experience of being on the diet. Which program will meet your need for pleasure? Which program allows enough flexibility that you're not forced to "cheat" from time to time? Which program adapts well to vacations, holidays, and parties? Which demands complex calculations? Which encourages you to eat a wide variety of food and provides the balanced nutrition you need for life?

Here's where so many people fail before they begin. By choosing a low-carb program that they can't possibly stay on for the rest of their lives, or which adds carbs in such a way as to set them up for cravings and eventual failure, dieters—understandably desperate to do *something*—find themselves repeating the same pattern of mistakes year after year.

This time we'd love to see you make a sane and realistic choice: one that fulfills your desire for comfortable, happy, rewarding, and long-lived success. As always, before you go any further, make certain that you follow your physician's recommendations with regard to the advisability of following any particular low-carb program.

No matter which program you move into, one thing is essential: that you take the time you need to get and prepare the food necessary to keep you happy and healthy.

Even though you think you know all about the low-carb program of your choice, we encourage you to read the book that describes it over again, cover to cover. You may discover surprising information you never realized was there!

Rereading the book that explains the fundamentals of the program you are intending to follow is more important than we can stress. Complete your rereading before you begin the program; take notes, work out the areas of concern. When you're finished, decide if it is still a doable plan for you.

Then sit down and write up a personal plan showing how you intend to move, in steps of one change only, from your current eating plan based on the completion of Day #7 into your new plan. If, for instance, your intended eating program involves giving up your Reward Meal and eating only low-carb food at every meal, you might give up one high-carb food per day as you move toward your final goal. If, on any day, you feel a great resistance to making any change, stay where you are and don't force yourself. Try again the next day.

If, day after day, you find yourself unwilling to incorporate the change, it may be that your intended program is too restrictive for you. The good news is that your choice is no longer between a program that is too restrictive and undisciplined high-carb eating. Remember that you were successful when you were allowed a balanced Reward Meal each day; you can still return to your eating at the end of Day #7, and with a bit of fine-tuning that we can provide, you can lose weight while still enjoying a daily treat.

So if you plan on moving to a different low-carb plan, get to know it well and move toward it in small steps. If, on the other hand, you find yourself unable or unwilling to make the changes required by a different plan, and while you are reacquainting yourself with the program of your choice, you can continue to eat as you were at the end of Day #7 of the 7-Day Jump-Start Plan, enjoying your (balanced!) Reward Meal every day.

If you stay at Day #7 for more than a few days, you'll need important tips to ensure your continued success. You can find them in *The Carbohydrate Addict's LifeSpan Program*, where— with your physician's approval—you can continue to enjoy a Reward Meal, continue to cut your cravings, continue your weight loss, and as the pounds drop off, move effortlessly, pleasurably, and consistently toward your ultimate weight goal.

PART II

Chapter 12

Five Vital Clues Low-Carb Diet Doctors Miss

Clue #1 : Saturated Fats Vs. High-Carbs: The Real Villain Is A Carbohydrate Act-Alike

You're probably aware of a battle that has been waging for years: "Eating foods high in fat makes you fat," claims one group of diet experts. "They do not!" challenges the opposition, equally expert and equally convinced they are right. "Foods that are high in *carbs* make you fat."

Each side, convinced they have the only handle on the truth, makes recommendations in keeping with their own beliefs, totally disregarding whatever new discoveries the other side claims to have made. Dieters, anxious to find a solution that works, are bombarded with the latest news, which often swings in one direction then the other.

So who's right? Do high carbs or high fats set off insulin responses that make us gain weight?

The answer is a resounding . . . both!

Either a diet high in carbs or one high in saturated fats (and/or trans fats) is likely to increase your insulin levels (or increase insulin resistance), which of course translates into more cravings and less weight loss (or none at all). It makes no sense to focus on one and ignore the other. It's like a competitive swimmer asking, "Which arm should I use for my strokes?" If you want to win the race, you had better use both.

The good news is that paying attention to both saturated fats and carbs in your diet is a lot easier than you think; it makes good health sense, and it is far more likely to produce results that keep you motivated and happy.* In addition, in the charts and pages that follow we'll help make it even simpler.

Remember that not all fats have been shown to raise insulin levels. From Dr. A. R. Folsom's study of over four thousand healthy, middle-aged adults, to Dr. K. D. Ward's research in the Normative Aging Study; from Dr. J. A. Marshall's study of over a thousand men and women from twenty to seventy-four years of age, to Dr. E. J. Mayer's study of nondiabetic women, the findings are the same: saturated fats increase insulin levels while unsaturated fats do not.

For the low-carb dieter, this discovery provides a powerful tool for keeping cravings and weight under control.

Even if the diet doctor who designed your low-carb program recommends foods high in saturated fats, by choosing only unsaturated fats (preferably monounsaturated fats), you may be able to avoid back-door insulin responses of which the diet doctor may not have been aware. A simple change from a low-carb protein that is high in saturated fat (such as a particularly fatty cut of beef) to one that is lower in saturated fat (such as fish, chicken, or a leaner cut of beef) can help reduce rebound cravings and keep your weight falling.

To avoid eating foods that could be slowing or stopping your weight loss, you'll need to know a bit about the differences among the types of fat. Don't worry, you won't need to know the biochemistry of lipids (thank goodness!), just a simple way of recognizing the good guys from the bad guys.

People sometimes throw around the phrase "trans fats" incorrectly, lumping them in with saturated fats when actually they're different. Trans fats, which are composed of trans fatty acids, can be as undesirable to the low-carb dieter as saturated fats and, in

---

*As always, check with your physician and follow his/her recommendations regarding the best eating program for your individual needs.

many cases, even more undesirable. By nature, they are unsaturated fats that have been chemically transformed from their normal room temperature liquid state into a solid. They may appear in ingredient labels as hydrogenated or partially hydrogenated fats. Food manufacturers like to include trans fats in your food (in place of margarine or butter) because these solid fats ensure that when opening the package, the consumer doesn't come face to face with some melted, oily mess. Trans fat may be most cost effective (that is, cheaper!) as well.

In addition, trans fats have a longer shelf life than other fats. So while they may have been sitting around for a very long time, the foods to which they have been added may still smell and feel fresh.

Although food manufacturers like to use trans fats, these fats have a darker side when it comes to your health and weight.

With each passing day, researchers are discovering new information about the impact of the different types of dietary fat. Anything we write may prove obsolete in a day! Still, the findings that came out of one of the best research studies to date are so powerful, we want to share them with you in hopes that these discoveries will help you make good choices in the years to come.

The Nurses' Health Study, published back in 1997, set the stage for hundreds of research studies that continue to validate this piece of landmark research. The study was published in the esteemed *New England Journal of Medicine* and conducted by Dr. Frank B. Hu and his colleagues at Harvard Medical College and Brigham and Women's Hospital, who followed over eighty thousand women for fourteen years.

Dr. Hu's team found that replacing only 5 percent of the women's daily caloric intake of carbohydrates with monounsaturated fats reduced their risk of heart disease by 19 percent. Replacing the same proportion of carbohydrates with polyunsaturated fats reduced the risk of heart disease by 38 percent. Dr. Hu's team also discovered that if they replaced only 2 percent of the women's daily caloric intake of carbohydrates with trans fats, there was a whopping 93 percent increase in heart disease!

> Replacing even a *tiny bit* of saturated fat
> with unsaturated fat may lower your risk
> of heart disease, motivate you to stay on
> your low-carb diet, and keep you losing
> weight—all at the same time.

By replacing one "bad" fat with a "good" one, major reductions in heart disease were achieved. Dr. Hu's team discovered that the simple swapping of fats, substituting only 5 percent of daily caloric intake in the form of saturated fats with the preferred unsaturated fats, reduced heart disease by nearly half, and trading only 2 percent of trans fats for unsaturated fats reduced heart disease by 53 percent. Dr. Hu's conclusion was simple: Replacing saturated and trans fats with polyunsaturated and mononounsaturated fats is more effective in reducing heart disease than reducing overall fat intake.

For you, the low-carb dieter, these findings as well as the studies that have since confirmed these early discoveries may mean a greater freedom to include "good" fat as part of your low-carb program, so long as you choose unsaturated fat as a safer alternative. As always, you must be guided by your physician's recommendations as new research adds to the field of knowledge and as your particular needs may require alternative choices.

In a Nutshell

In keeping with your physician's recommendations, choose low-carb proteins that are lower in saturated fat. Differences in total fat content among animal products are generally accounted for by saturated fat. Therefore, when comparing different cuts of beef, poultry, or cheese, using total fat content as your guide works well.

It's important to use a fat counter with easy-to-read pages, like the chart below from our *Carbohydrate Addict's Fat Counter.*

MEATS*
(sample partial chart)

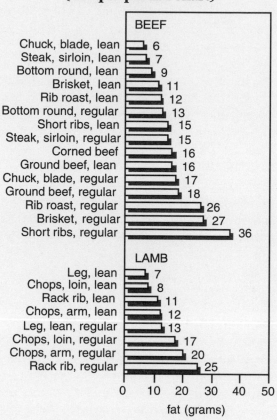

BEEF

Cut	fat (grams)
Chuck, blade, lean	6
Steak, sirloin, lean	7
Bottom round, lean	9
Brisket, lean	11
Rib roast, lean	12
Bottom round, regular	13
Short ribs, lean	15
Steak, sirloin, regular	15
Corned beef	16
Ground beef, lean	16
Chuck, blade, regular	17
Ground beef, regular	18
Rib roast, regular	26
Brisket, regular	27
Short ribs, regular	36

LAMB

Cut	fat (grams)
Leg, lean	7
Chops, loin, lean	8
Rack rib, lean	11
Chops, arm, lean	12
Leg, lean, regular	13
Chops, loin, regular	17
Chops, arm, regular	20
Rack rib, regular	25

fat (grams)

Counts are based on 3-ounce servings.

Charts with easy-to-read graphics can help you make smart low-fat choices by comparing the fat content of a variety of proteins or showing differences in fat content among cuts of the same type of meat (which can vary by as much as 600 percent!).

With such quick information in hand, you're far less likely to let fat sneak up on you and ruin all your good work.

*Page 125, *The Carbohydrate Addict's Fat Counter,* by Drs. Rachael and Richard Heller.

Labels with a Twist

If you think you have it all straight (and we hope you do), some food manufacturers have added yet another twist that is sure to keep you on your toes.

Here's how it goes: In order to make an unsaturated fat into a trans fat, extra hydrogen atoms are pumped into the unsaturated fat. This is called the hydrogenation process. When hydrogen atoms are added, the formerly unsaturated fat is turned into a saturated fat, obliterating any benefits it had as a polyunsaturated fat.

Though both descriptions are technically correct, food manufacturers prefer to use the term "trans unsaturated fat" instead of just plain "trans fat," perhaps because the former contains the word "unsaturated." Though "trans unsaturated fat" sounds like it's good for you, it most certainly is not.

Question: When Is an Unsaturated Fat Not an Unsaturated Fat?

Answer: When it has been changed into a trans fat.

Understanding the difference between an unsaturated fat and a trans fat may surprise you or make you mad (or both). We hope, in addition, it arms you with the information you need to take better care of yourself.

Both saturated fats and trans fats tend to be solids or semi-solids at room temperature. Some typical sources of saturated fat include butter, shortening, coconut oil, palm oil, and the fat from meats. Unsaturated fats, on the other hand, are generally liquid at room temperature. Examples are olive oil, vegetable oil, and peanut oil.

Trans fats can be found in vegetable shortenings and many margarines and, as we said before, are often included in packaged cookies, crackers, and other baked goods. In addition, they are often used in making French fries.

FAST FAT FACTS TO GO

The fats and oils you eat contain different amounts of all types of fat: trans fatty acids (that make up trans fats), saturated fat, polyunsaturated fat, and monounsaturated fat. The fats are listed below according to their highest concentrations of a particular kind of fat.

This chart will help you spot the fats that are least likely to raise your insulin levels, increase your cravings, and slow your weight loss, and which are more most likely to.

LEAST likely to raise insulin levels	HIGH IN MONO-UNSATURATED FATS	HIGH IN POLY-UNSATURATED FATS	HIGH IN SATURATED FATS	HIGH IN TRANS FATTY ACIDS	MOST likely to raise insulin levels
	olive oil canola oil peanut oil	safflower oil soybean oil corn oil sunflower oil sesame oil cottonseed oil omega-3 oils	butter fat beef fat lard milk fat coconut oil chicken fat palm oil cocoa butter	vegetable shortening, hydrogenated fats, some margarines	

REMEMBER: Trans fats (and the trans fatty acids they're made of) are sometimes listed on ingredient labels as trans unsaturated fats, although processing has removed any of their former unsaturated-fat-related benefits.

At this time, trans fats appear to be the most insulin stimulating of all fats. Trans fats (and trans fatty acids) may also be listed on ingredient labels as hydrogenated fats or partially hydrogenated fats. By any name, trans fatty acids do not appear to be good for your heart health and, because of the insulin release they may set in motion, may make it more difficult for you to stay on your low-carb diet and lose weight.

Future research may produce changes in our understanding of the relationship of dietary lipids to heart health and weight loss, but for now most researchers are recommending monoun-saturated fats and/or polyunsaturated fats in place of saturated fats and trans fats.

If your low-carb program recommends saturated fats and/or does not limit the amount of saturated fats you eat, we suggest that you reconsider that recommendation, speak with your physi-cian, and perhaps substitute monounsaturated and/or polyunsat-urated fats in place of saturated fats and trans fats.

Clue #2: Sugar Substitutes: A Second Carbohydrate Act-Alike

We could easily divide low-carb dieters into two groups based on the following question: "Do you use sugar substitutes on a regular basis?" Among those who do *not* use sugar substitutes regularly, we could expect to find the majority successfully los-ing weight, without cravings. Among those who do, however, we could expect a troubled history of intermittent cravings, fatigue, lack of motivation, on-again-off-again dieting interspersed with cheating, weight-loss slowdowns and plateaus.

> Whether in the form of a "natural" or artificial sweetener, sugar substitutes may signal the body to release high levels of insulin.

In our years of research and teaching at one of the nation's top medical schools, we have seen clear evidence that one of the most powerful triggers for insulin release is one that most low-carb dieters never think about: sugar substitutes.

Whether in the form of a "natural" or an artificial sweetener, sugar substitutes may signal the body to release high levels of insulin. Wrapped up in little blue packs or pink packs, referred to by this brand name or that, they seem to act upon the body in similar ways.

We have found that if you are sensitive to carbohydrates, sugar substitutes can raise your insulin levels, increase your insulin resistance, and/or cause unexpected blood sugar swings.

> When it sees, smells, or tastes
> sugar substitute, your body can
> "think" it is getting real sugar.

The reason for the power of sugar substitutes to play havoc with your insulin levels, cravings, and weight loss is simple. When you consume foods or drinks that are naturally sweet, the carbohydrates in that food or drink are turned into simple sugar.

On seeing, smelling, or tasting the food or drink sweetened with a sugar substitute, your body perceives it as real sugar. In order to transport the anticipated sugar to muscle and organ cells to be used as fuel, insulin surges into your bloodstream.

Once there, the insulin finds that no sugar has been metabolized from the sugar-free food you have just eaten. Needing to "couple" with sugar, it may pull much of the blood sugar out of your bloodstream, signaling your liver to store it away as fat.

Although you ate or drank only sugarless foods, the sweet taste (sometimes six hundred times as sweet as sugar) has left you with high insulin levels and blood sugar swings that are quite likely to set off intense cravings for carbohydrates and start your body into a fat-making cycle.

Many low-carb dieters, experiencing the cravings for carbohydrates that go along with low blood sugar swings and high insulin levels, reach again for drinks or foods sweetened with a sugar substitute, and begin the entire process again. Soon they find themselves in an endless cycle of emotional ups and downs, suffering cravings, weakness, and irritability, and—although they may fight off the urge to cheat—still see little real progress in their weight loss.

Weary and confused as to why they are not doing better when they have been "so good," many low-carb dieters give up, never knowing that the real culprit was right in front of them in that innocent sugar substitute they had always assumed was their friend.

When our bodies evolved a few million years ago, sugar substitutes did not exist. Our bodies were made to handle "real" sugar and to this day treat anything that tastes sweet as if it contains real sugar. There is no way around it; if something tastes sweet, your body assumes it contains sugar and releases insulin— the hunger hormone, the fat-making hormone.

Many low-carb gurus favor one or another of the sugar substitutes, recommending some and telling you to avoid others (often without a great deal of explanation as to the reason for the distinction). Other low-carb diet doctors indicate that sugar substitutes should be avoided "when possible," but fail to explain their somewhat veiled position. We fear it is because, in many cases, they are afraid to say what some weight-loss professionals suspect: that sugar substitutes have ruined more low-carb diets than lack of willpower, loss of motivation, and chocolate cake put together.

So while you thought you were being so good, you may have been so bad—to yourself and your chances for weight-loss success.

Are You Addicted to Diet Drinks?

Try these questions on for size:

Do you find that an hour or two after having a diet drink, you crave more of the same?

When you thought a diet soda would do, do you find yourself reaching for a snack or sandwich or something sweet to eat with it?

Do you tell yourself it's a good thing that you drink diet so-das because they help you save calories (though you sometimes eat less when you don't have them)?

Do you get a special feeling of satisfaction when you take your first sip?

Did you find the taste of diet sodas unpleasant when you first tried them but now find the taste acceptable? Or do you still dislike the taste but drink the diet soda anyway?

Do you ever think you might be addicted to diet drinks?

Does the thought of giving them up make you uncomfortable?

Is a meal or snack just "not the same" without a diet soda?

"Yes" answers to any of these questions indicate that you may be experiencing an addictive response to sugar substitutes. The greater the number of "yes" answers, the greater the possibility that an addiction to diet sodas may be contributing to your low-carb diet problems, cravings, and weight-loss plateaus.

> We have found that, for many low-carb dieters, avoiding sugar substitutes can make the difference between success and failure.

We have found that, for many low-carb dieters, avoiding sugar substitutes can make the difference between success and failure. While many low-carb diet doctors will tell you to go ahead and indulge, we'll ask you to listen to your own body. If that first sip of a diet soda gives you intense pleasure, a feeling of "Whew! I made it"; if within an hour or two after drinking a diet soda you feel irritable, headachy, or tired; or if drinking diet soda makes you want to reach for the nearest high-carb treat, consider that, contrary to what many may have told you, for you sugar free is no free ride.

Freedom by Preference

If giving up sugar substitutes is something you'd like to try but if you are unsure you can do it—or how to do it—we have a suggestion that has worked well.

Instead of imposing more demands on yourself (you probably already have enough people telling you what to do), we suggest you try the following for the next few days: whenever you consider having a diet soda or a dessert, gum, or mint that has been sweetened with sugar substitutes, *ask* yourself if you could possibly do without it.

Don't *push* yourself or *demand* that you give up a diet soda that you really want. On the other hand, if you're drinking a diet soda out of habit or because it happens to be there, consider choosing a glass of cold water, seltzer, or unsweetened iced tea instead. Make the choice a matter of preference. If you really want it, have it. If you can live without it, decide to pass it up.

We have discovered that with this approach, you'll find yourself choosing the sugar substitute less and less often. We stress that you *ask* yourself to forgo the sugar substitutes for a few days, not *demand* strict and unconditional compliance.

A simple request to yourself to cut down, cut back, and then let go of sugar substitutes will often go a great deal further than you might imagine. In four days, as your insulin responses and blood sugar levels come into balance, you may experience a rise in confidence and a feeling of freedom that will help ensure your continuing success. What might have been a challenge in the past will become part of your new way of living (and eating!).

Clue #3: Glutamates: A Third Carbohydrate Act-Alike

MSG (monosodium glutamate) as well as other glutamates can appear in food naturally, but food manufacturers now routinely add glutamates to enhance the flavor of foods. We have noticed that among many low-carb dieters, in particular those who are especially sensitive to carbohydrates, glutamates can bring about an addictive response—one that pushes the dieter to consume more of the glutamate-enhanced foods or to eat them more often.

Without knowing it, low-carb dieters may be selecting brands that contain higher levels of added glutamates, not because these foods taste better or because they satisfy them more fully, but rather because they are experiencing an addictive response to the glutamates in them.

Food manufacturers have long known that we have glutamate receptors in our taste buds. These receptors drive us to seek out and consume foods that contain glutamates, even when we cannot actually identify the taste of the glutamates and don't know when we're consuming them.

Glutamates seem to enhance other tastes as well as the sensation of taste in general—but at a price.

> Glutamates can be hidden in our foods under
> a wide variety of names. By any name they
> can still spell high levels of insulin.

Of most importance to low-carb dieters is the discovery that glutamates added to foods can cause the body to release insulin. As Dr. N. A. Togiyama and Dr. A. Adachi reported in the medical journal *Physiological Behavior*, the application of monosodium glutamate to the tongues of animals will cause them to release high levels of insulin within three minutes.

Three minutes! Unsuspecting low-carb dieters may never know why, after eating something that tastes especially satisfying, they can't stop.

> Even as we write these pages,
> food manufacturers are finding new
> ways to include glutamates in your food—
> without your ever knowing it.

Glutamates are categorized as excitotoxins, that is, they cause the injury or death of cells by stimulation. While scientists are still exploring the long-term effects of glutamates, food manufacturers forge ahead, finding new ways to include them in your food—without your ever knowing it. Food in cans and packages that do not appear to have changed may now contain one or more newly added glutamates.

One of the most obvious examples is within the canned fish industry. Several years ago, when tuna manufacturers felt the pressure to replace oil-packed tuna with a water-packed variety, they faced a major dilemma. While consumers clearly preferred the water pack for health reasons, this variety was decidedly less tasty than its oil-based predecessor. Food manufacturers solved their problem by adding free glutamates (chemicals that are very similar in structure to monosodium glutamate) which not only enhanced the flavor of the water-packed tuna but also did not appear to the consumer to be as "unhealthy" as oil.

Added under one of a dozen names, one or more glutamates began appearing in the ingredient labels of virtually every major brand of canned tuna—though the *front* of the can still sported the familiar "tuna in spring water" label. Unsuspecting consumers never knew—nor do most realize to this day—that while they were being so "good" on their low-carb diets, they were actually ingesting chemicals that could be interfering with their best efforts to control their eating and promote their weight loss.

While it is relatively easy to avoid many food additives by reading the ingredient label, it is much more difficult to detect the addition of glutamates, which may be included under so many names that to really know what you're eating, you have to compare the nutritional label with the long list on page 127.

To make matters even more difficult for the unsuspecting consumer, many of the names used for glutamates may sound very benign, even healthy, including "broth" and "natural flavors."

Low-carb dieters, assuming that something labeled "natural flavors" should not cause concern, may never imagine that so healthy-sounding an ingredient might come back to haunt them in the form of cravings and weight gain. After all, they reason, if it's natural, what can be bad about it? Well, cyanide, arsenic, and dirt are also natural, but no one would want them added to their food.

Still, the deceptively innocent image of anything called "natural flavors" or "broth" is difficult to counter.

Only a few of the low-salt, low-calorie varieties of canned tuna contain no glutamates. You can spot the glutamate-free brands because the ingredient list on the label (not the starburst on the front of the can) reads: tuna, water (and nothing else).

Look at a can of tuna. If the ingredient list
includes broth or hydrolyzed protein, it
probably contains glutamates.

While manufacturers may not lie, some don't always tell the entire truth. When we called the top two manufacturers of canned tuna fish, we were told that no monosodium glutamate had been added to their tuna. When we asked specifically if *free* glutamates were added, both companies confirmed our suspicion. Though they knew that, for our purposes, there was almost no difference between free glutamates and monosodium glutamate, both companies refused to admit the presence of this additive until they were forced to do so.

When scientists want obese lab animals for
experiments, they often get rats that were
made fat by being fed MSG.

When added to food, glutamates can have powerful consequences. In laboratory animals they break down the muscle fiber and cause brain damage. Did you know that scientists who want obese lab animals for experimentation call the supply house and ask for MSG-fattened rats? The rats become obese simply by eating monosodium glutamate in their feed!

So while some may claim that there is nothing wrong with glutamates, we say if you are trying to lose weight (especially on a low-carb diet), stay away from MSG and all other added glutamates. These chemicals may increase your insulin levels, slow down your weight loss, and make you so hungry that you can hardly be expected to stay on your low-carb diet—all without your ever knowing why.

Whenever low-carb dieters tell us that they are having repeated problems getting on or staying on their plan, or when they report a sudden jump in cravings or in their weight, we ask them to check the ingredient labels on the foods they've been eating. Almost invariably they discover the source of their problem in the many glutamates they have been consuming under a host of names. When these foods are substituted with brands that do not contain glutamates, or with fresh foods, a renewed sense of calm and control often returns to the dieter within a few days.

> At least one-third of all restaurant meals
> contain added glutamates, but you can easily
> avoid them when eating at home.

Added glutamates appear to be more of a problem for low-carb dieters than naturally occurring glutamates. Unfortunately, if you eat out, you probably can't avoid them. At least one-third of all the food you eat in restaurants contains added glutamates, which explains why, in part, some of us tend to put on a pound or two after eating out.

You are almost forced to put up with glutamates in order to live a normal life, but when you have a choice such as when you buy food in grocery stores, it's important to read the label and, as much as possible, avoid food with added glutamates.

Food manufacturers can add glutamates by including any of the following ingredients:

Anything enzyme modified	Hydrolyzed soy protein
Anything fermented	Malt extract
Anything protein fortified	Maltodextrin
Anything ultra pasteurized	Natural flavors (flavoring)
Autolyzed yeast	Pectin
Barley malt	Plant protein extract
Broth	Potassium glutamate
Bouillon	Sodium caseinate
Calcium caseinate	Soy protein
Carrageen	Soy sauce
Flavoring	Stock
Gelatin	Textured protein
Hydrolyzed oat flour	Whey protein
Hydrolyzed vegetable protein	Yeast extract
Hydrolyzed plant protein	Yeast food

You can't live in fear of added glutamates, so unless you want to grow all of your own food and cook everything from scratch, you have to tolerate some. But when you can, it would be wise to avoid them.

Glutamates may be the "pull" to your
favorite restaurant or food.

If you find yourself unexplainably *drawn* to a certain restaurant or a certain brand of food, if it gives you a strong sense of pleasure, or almost a sense of relief, when you take the first bite, or as it has been described, if it gives you a "hit," even though you know it's not the finest in culinary cuisine, you may be surprised to know you're feeling the effects of the added glutamates.

A rose by any other name may smell as sweet, but glutamates by any name do not.

Clue #4: The Frequency Factor Offers Freedom For Life

Have you ever seen a movie in which the hero, on the trail of the bad guy, seeks him out at a certain location while you, the audience, know that the bad guy isn't there? While the good guy rushes madly in the wrong direction, the bad guy makes his way to the jewels, girl, detonation device, or escape. You sit by watching the movie play out, hoping that in the end, the good guy will see the error of his ways and get back on the right track. Well, we love happy endings (in movies and in life) and watching people focus on only one of the carbohydrate-related obesity-inducing factors while ignoring the other, perhaps more important factor is not easy.

> Low-carb dieters are starting to find that counting carb grams and eating low-carb foods are not the whole answer.

We have all watched as dieters moved from the era of calorie counting to fat gram counting to carb gram counting. While at first each of these approaches to weight loss seemed to hold the answer, in time each failed to help the dieter take it off and keep it off. Just like those dieters of years ago, low-carb dieters today are starting to find that counting carb grams and eating low-carb foods is not the whole answer.

"I just couldn't continue to live like that," we were told by one low-carb dieter after another. "There has to come a time when you can eat like a normal person. But when I do, I start to put the weight right back on. There's got to be a better way."

There is a better way and we've been doing it successfully and helping millions of other people to do it for for more than twenty years. Although it's clear that carbohydrates hold an essential key to cravings and weight gain, the *amount* of carbohydrate you eat is not the only factor.

While focusing on the amount of high-carb foods they eat, unsuspecting low-carb dieters may be missing an even more important contributor to weight gain: the Frequency Factor. While it is true that the amount of carbohydrates you eat within a given time helps determine whether you lose or gain weight, it is equally true that how often you eat high-carb foods can have just as powerful an effect (or, in some cases, an even greater influence).

Here's what happens inside your body: When you see, smell, think of a high-carb food, or when you take your first bite, your body immediately releases insulin. Just as your body produces saliva to help break up the food that's coming in, your body produces insulin to help metabolize incoming carbohydrates.

Insulin is needed to open up the cells in your body to allow the high-carb food (which has been changed into blood sugar, that is, glucose) to pass from your bloodstream into the cells. The cells in your brain and the rest of your nervous system get nourished first, then your other organs and muscles.

> In order to lose fat, you have to get your
> body *out* of its Saving Mode and
> into a Spending Mode.

Put in basic terms, this energy moves in one direction, from the bloodstream into the cells of the muscles and organs. Whatever blood sugar remains once the muscles and organs have had their fill is turned into blood fat. The remaining insulin in the blood now signals the fat cells to open up to let in the blood fat, for storage in the fat cells.

So when your insulin levels are high, you are in a Saving Mode, moving energy into cells to be used as needed or, when no longer needed, to be stored. As long as insulin levels remain high, your body is on a one-way street, with energy flowing into the fat cells.

In order to lose fat from your fat cells, you have to get your body out of its Saving Mode and into a Spending Mode. As the pounds continue to drop, you want to stay in the Spending Mode for as long as possible, while still taking in the nutrition you need to stay healthy and the pleasure you need to stay motivated. Fortunately, that's not difficult.

Now here's the key point: There are *two* ways (at least) to keep insulin levels low enough to help you stay in a Spending Mode. The first way is to keep carbohydrate intake very low. This way of losing weight is well known to every low-carb dieter.

It's all so simple, you've been told. To lose weight you eat only low-carb foods. As long as your body does not sense that you have eaten food that contains carbs of any significance, it will have no need to put out a surge of insulin; lower levels of insulin translate into the spending of fat from your fat cells. Sounds logical. At first, anyway.

The problem is, you can't stay on a low-carb diet indefinitely; you need carbohydrate-rich foods in order to stay alive and, some say, to make life worth living. Adding any sort of high-carb food back into the diet is where the difficulty occurs for most low-carb dieters.

The second way to keep insulin levels low is to eat high-carb foods no more than once a day. Apparently, the more often you eat high-carb foods, the more often you release insulin, with each successive insulin release being greater than the previous one. So the more often you eat high-carb foods throughout the day, the greater the surge of insulin each time, and the longer you remain in a Saving Mode.

What is of most importance to the low-carb dieter is the reverse of this finding: when you have not eaten high-carb foods for a while, your insulin levels drop. Your muscles and organs, no longer flooded with insulin and blood sugar, begin to run out of energy and the flow of energy is reversed; it comes out of the fat cells in order to resupply the lagging organs and muscles. The released energy from the fat cells (blood fat) is turned back into blood sugar and used to fuel cells in the muscles and organs.

> Nature has built a sort of "safety switch" into
> the system that allows us a little leeway.

The longer insulin levels remain low (because you haven't eaten high-carb foods), the longer your body has a chance to release fat from the fat cells and burn it up. Each pound you lose is proof positive that your body has remained long enough in a Spending Mode to burn up some of its fat stores.

Nature has built a sort of "safety switch" into the system that allows us a little leeway within this incredibly balanced machine we call our bodies. This safety switch alone can spell success to the low-carb dieter. When you have not eaten high-carb foods for a while and then indulge in a high-carb meal, the amount of insulin you release will usually be *far less* than if this meal followed another recent high-carb meal.

Once again, whether you lose weight, stay at the same weight, or gain weight is determined not only by the amount of high-carb food you eat but also by *how often* you eat it.

We refer to this natural phenomenon as the "Frequency Factor," and most low-carb diet doctors seem unaware of its power. When you take advantage of this natural phenomenon, you get to have your cake and lose weight too.

> By using the Frequency Factor to your
> advantage, you can add high-carb foods back
> into your diet while continuing to lose weight.

When you decrease the number of times each day that you eat high-carb foods, *even if the total intake of high-carb food for the day is the same,* you can keep your insulin levels lower and keep your body in a Spending Mode for longer periods of time. Longer periods of Spending mean greater weight loss and fewer cravings. (Your body doesn't need you to take in food while it's busy spending the energy you have already stored.) By taking advantage of the Frequency Factor, when you add high-carb foods back into your diet, as long as you do so less frequently, you can still enjoy the foods you love without seeing a jump in your cravings or your weight.

For more information on the Frequency Factor, see Day #5 of the 7-Day Jump Start Plan. For additional help in incorporating high-carb foods into your daily eating plan, see *The Carbohydrate Addict's LifeSpan Program.*

Clue #5: Beating The Insulin Countdown: Eating Toward Your Carbs

Suppose you discovered a way of eating that allowed people on low-carb diets to reduce cravings and increase weight loss without changing *what* they ate, only *the order in which they ate it?* In addition, imagine that, as far as you could see, not one of the low-carb diets so popular in this country had ever included this information?

Well, that's where we stand and why we think it's so important that you know what we know, even if they don't know . . . you know? It's our way of sending you a personal letter that says, "Listen, we've got some great news for you! It's easy, it doesn't mean giving up anything, and—best of all—it can work wonders!"

Chances are, you have never been told that the *order* in which you eat your food can make the difference.

So here's what we've learned: we have found that for you to achieve the most weight loss and have the fewest cravings, it's important to eat toward your carbs. That means that, in any meal that contains foods that are not low-carb (whether it's your daily Reward Meal on our Carbohydrate Addict's LifeSpan Program or any meal to which you have added carbs in keeping with your low-carb program), you should start the meal by eating the foods that are lowest in carbohydrates and finish with the foods that are highest.

The doctors behind most low-carb diets put limits on *what* you can eat and restrictions on *how much* you can eat, but chances are you have never been told that the *order* in which you eat your food can make the difference between an effortless and successful weight-loss experience and one that is not.

Eating toward your carbs may seem like an odd recommendation, but its powerful and positive benefits are simple and important. We believe that this easy and essential strategy can be so important to weight loss and weight maintenance that, although we touch on it in Day #4 of the 7–Day Jump–Start Plan, we've added more information here. In this way, when the garlic bread (that you can have later in your meal) or the chocolate cake (with which you can finish off your Reward Meal) tempt you by whispering "Come on, just one bite," you'll be armed and ready to say, "Hold on. I'll be with you in a minute."

Working *With* Your Body Really Works!

Whenever you eat high-carbohydrate foods, your body releases insulin in two waves. Scientists call this the biphasic or two phase release of insulin. The first wave, or phase, starts within a few minutes of tasting, seeing, smelling, or thinking about high-carbohydrate food.

You have probably experienced this first wave of insulin release after having taken a bite or two of food. Suddenly you find you're hungrier than you thought you were. This quick jump in hunger, as well as the intense pleasure the food gives you, can be proof positive of your body's first wave of insulin.

The first wave is basically an on-off mechanism. In other words, your body releases insulin in one surge as soon as it gets the signal to "let 'er flow." The amount of insulin that is released depends on how much and how often you have eaten high-carbohydrate foods in the previous twelve to twenty hours. The less often you've eaten them, the less insulin your body is likely to release in this first wave.

When you start off your meal with high-carb
foods, you set off the Insulin Countdown.

So here you are about to eat a nice portion of high-carb food
in keeping with your program, and at the first taste your body
releases the first surge of insulin.

"Well, so what?" you might ask us. "After all, I'm *allowed* a bit
of high-carb (or high*er*-carb) food. I've moved out of the begin-
ner's phase of the program and I've been 'good' all day. So if my
body's about to release insulin, what can I do about it?"

The answer is . . . plenty!

With that first bite of high-carb food, your body begins an Insulin Countdown. It's keeping track of the approximately sixty
minutes before it will release a second wave of insulin.

After about an hour, your body checks to see if you are still
eating high-carbs. If you are, it assumes that you will need more
insulin and releases a backup load of the fat-saving substance.
This second surge of insulin is your body's way of making sure
that you have all the insulin you need to use the carbohydrates
you are eating. The whole system makes a lot of sense . . . if
you're a caveman!

Imagine, for a moment, that it's several hundred thousand
years ago. You're a caveman wandering the land in search of
food that, hopefully, will not fight back. You come across a clus-
ter of trees bearing fruit, tiny, wrinkled, and half-rotten perhaps
but fruit nonetheless.

Hoping this unknown fruit will not poison you, you begin to
eat it in great handfuls. It tastes wonderful! You've just released
the first wave of insulin. Since you haven't eaten anything but
meat and leaves for a long time, the amount of insulin in the
first wave is not very high. Based on your recent past meals, your
body didn't expect you to be eating high carbs. Now, here's the
most important point: with that first delicious bite, your body
begins its Insulin Countdown.

Sixty minutes later, your body checks back to make certain it
gave you enough insulin to handle the meal at hand. If you are

still eating high-carb foods (which you are, since there's plenty of fruit and you have no idea where your next meal is coming from), your body puts out a second insulin release.

> By delaying your high-carb foods *just a bit*,
> you can beat the Insulin Countdown.

The low-carb dieter's ability to significantly reduce the second surge of insulin or to avoid it entirely is why the eating-toward-your-carbs strategy works so well. In our research, we have found that by shortening the length of time you eat high-carbohydrate foods within a meal, you can beat the Insulin Countdown. That is *not*, we repeat, *not* to say that you eat quickly or that you shovel down your food.

In order to shorten the time during which you eat high-carb foods, you simply begin them later in the meal, that is, closer to the end. By holding on and waiting until later in the meal before that first bite of high-carb food, you can reduce the powerful effect of a second surge of insulin.

An increased second wave of insulin can send you into a Saving Mode that will help store that meal away in your fat cells rather than burn it up. While in the Saving Mode, your body is busy converting the blood sugar from your recent meal into blood fat, storing it in your fat cells and leaving you with more fat but less energy to keep going. With less blood sugar, after about two hours, you'll probably find yourself hungry once more, your body urging you to start the whole process over again.

> The longer you keep eating past the point of
> satisfaction, the *less* satisfied you feel.
> That's your second release of insulin.

Chances are you have experienced this second phase of insulin release at times when meals continued for extended periods of time; at leisurely restaurant dinners, family celebrations or holidays, for example. At these times, you may have eaten until you were satisfied, only to find that as you continued to eat, you became *less* satisfied than you were before. The more food you consumed, the less satisfaction you experienced. You might have eaten to the point of being uncomfortable (until you felt like you were bursting) while at the same time feeling less "finished" than you had earlier in the meal.

This is usually evidence of insulin's second wave reaching its peak about an hour after the first bite of high-carb food. It's the reason why we strongly recommend that in order to keep cravings down and weight falling, you eat toward your carbs.

> To eat the foods you love without guilt or fear . . . it's one of the great pleasures in life.

You will find an easy explanation of how eating toward your carbs works and a sample menu in Day #4 of the 7-Day Jump-Start Plan. The Guidelines you find there will help clarify what works and how. For some help in eating toward your carbs at restaurants, see Chapter 16. We think you'll enjoy some of the real life solutions we've come up with. You may even think of a couple of your own.

After all, one of the great pleasures in life is eating the foods you love without the guilt and fear that so many of you have lived with for so long. You've got it coming, and we'll help you do it.

Chapter 13

HIDDEN CARBS . . . WAITING TO POUNCE

"But I stuck to my diet *perfectly*. I never ate *anything* I wasn't supposed to and I just stopped losing weight."

"It worked for me in the beginning, then it stopped. Now when I eat *exactly* what I was eating before, I don't lose any weight . . . and I'm hungry all the time too."

> When you stop losing weight and you don't know why . . .

We've heard it a thousand times, maybe ten thousand, and each time we hear it, we cringe. So many people, thinking they are being so "good," never realize that a harmless looking food or ingredient—something they'd never dream could be important—is wiping out the good effects of their hard work and sacrifice.

How many others think they've failed, or that their diet has failed them, when something as simple as the coffee creamer they considered to be a tiny indulgence or a simple drink or dessert they thought was low-carb was spiking their insulin levels as much as any rich dessert or decadent indulgence.

Even the most experienced dieter can be fooled by hidden

carbs. How many people, for instance, would ever guess that two stalks of broccoli contain as many carbohydrates as a chocolate-covered ice cream bar? We are *not* saying you should go out and eat ice cream instead of your vegetables, and certainly broccoli contains fiber (among other good things) that's important for your health. On the other hand, if you're extremely sensitive to carbohydrates, even something as good for you as broccoli can signal your body to release insulin and make it harder to keep losing weight.

> Two stalks of broccoli contain
> as many carbohydrates as a
> chocolate-covered ice cream bar.*

This comparison is offered only as one of many examples we can make to illustrate the point that the carb counts of different foods may surprise you. We hope that the facts you'll find in the pages that follow will arm you against assumptions you may never have known you were making, and deceptions (intentional and otherwise) that others may be aiming in your direction.

Carb-Myth #1:
Drinks Don't Matter *That* Much!

Americans have come to believe that, with the exception of some alcoholic drinks, what you drink isn't going to make you fat. It's an odd idea, clearly wrong, but one that sticks.

While most of us know that fruit juice derives 100 percent of its calories from sugar, it still seems like such a "good" thing to

---

*While we've used this example to illustrate the point that the carb counts of many foods may surprise you, it is only one of many examples you may find in a wide variety of products from many food manufacturers.

drink that few people consider it the high-carb insulin booster
that it is.

> America's best-selling bottled teas are
> loaded with more carbs
> than you can imagine.

Tea is another of the "healthful" drinks that dieters tend to
overlook as a typical hiding place for carbs. One of America's
best-selling bottled teas* is loaded with carbs. While dieters may
be enjoying their green tea, they may also be fortifying themselves with sugars—to the equivalent of more than four teaspoons of sugar per eight-ounce glass and the equivalent of more
than ten teaspoons of sugar per twenty-ounce bottle.

Although a starburst on the label says the tea contains green
tea and honey, the ingredient list also notes high fructose corn
syrup as its second ingredient and in greater proportion than the
honey.*

One of the other teas made by the same company appears to
be even higher in carbs. Each eight-ounce glass of one of their
specialty teas* contains the equivalent of nearly seven teaspoons
of sugar, while the entire twenty-ounce bottle contains the equivalent of more than seventeen teaspoons of sugar.

> Plateaus broken,
> just by changing your drink.

We've known low-carb dieters, stuck at plateaus for months,
who started losing weight again by simply replacing their bottled

---

*While we've used this example to illustrate the point that the carb counts of many
foods may surprise you, it is only one of many examples you may find in a wide variety of products from many food manufacturers.

tea or other beverage with a homemade variety. On seeing a new weight loss, some became angry at all the time and effort they'd wasted by not realizing they were drinking their carbs. Others were thrilled to be losing again when they thought they'd never see the scale budge. Most confessed they knew the tea tasted too good to be sugar-free, but since it was *only* tea they thought it wouldn't matter all that much.

Be sure not to substitute one problem with another. If you want to keep your insulin levels down and your weight dropping, you'll do far better by making your own unsweetened tea than by buying the "unsweetened" packaged or bottled variety that is loaded with sugar substitutes. Remember that while sugar substitutes may contain almost no carbs, they can signal the body to release insulin almost like sugar does. So while you're not consuming a high-carb drink, per se, your body thinks you are and sends out an insulin surge. So if it tastes sweet, you might want to think twice (or three times) before having it.*

> Why else would flavored
> coffees taste so good?

Keep your eyes open when you reach for that cup of coffee as well. There's a reason why flavored coffees taste great! Most of them contain alcohol and/or sugar that can turn your plain cup of no-carb coffee into a well of carbohydrates (or Carbohydrate Act-Alikes).

Even if your favorite hazelnut or mocha flavoring doesn't contain a significant amount of high-carb ingredients, it can fool your body into thinking it's getting something sweet.

Little additions like coffee creamers can take a plain, carbohydrate-free cup of coffee and turn it into a high-carb insulin spiker. A little "treat" of French vanilla creamer in your cof-

---

*For more information on sugar substitutes and their effect on insulin, cravings, and weight-loss plateaus or slowdowns, see the chapter "Five Vital Clues Low-Carb Diet Doctors Miss."

fee can contain one teaspoon of sugar for every two teaspoons of creamer. If you're looking at total carbs, the count is even worse: three-quarters of every spoonful of creamer is made up of carbs.

> A tiny change can make a big difference in your weight loss.

If you sip the coffee slowly and prolong the insulin release, you're more likely to put on more weight (or lose weight more slowly) than if you consumed the same number of carbs in an out-and-out piece of high-carb food. The truth is, your body knows where the carbs are hidden and even if they look innocent to you, even if you pretend you don't know they're there, your body does.

On the other hand, the good news is that if you're not sure what's keeping the weight on (or the cravings strong), it may be that a small change can make a big difference in your weight loss.

Carb-Myth #2:
You Should Have Seen What I *Didn't* Eat!

There's an odd thinking that accompanies many kinds of diets but seems especially pronounced when it comes to low-carb eating. It goes something like this: I could have really done damage to my diet by eating something *really* high in carbs. Instead, I ate something that wasn't quite so bad. So I should be praised rather than chastised.

Okay, we don't want to admit how many times that fuzzy logic has crossed our own minds. We all know it doesn't make sense. Still, it seems as if we should be rewarded for being . . . so good!

Of course, the truth is that diets don't work that way. Whether you go one inch over the edge of the cliff or ten feet, you're still looking at a hard fall. Physical reality doesn't give you credit for being almost right. As long as you put high-carbs into your mouth, your body doesn't care what you *didn't* eat. And here's the funniest part. We've discovered that the food you "allowed" yourself in place of the super high-carb food you resisted is often just as bad (or worse)!

Here's a typical example: Ianna, thirty-eight, was recently divorced and new on the job in a real-estate office. Within the first week, she became the designated "gopher," sent to fill everyone's mid-morning coffee break requests at the nearby national donut outlet.* Committed to staying on her low-carb plan, Ianna mustered her self-control and refused to let herself order even one donut while organizing and transporting all of her coworkers' tempting goodies.

As compensation for being so "good," she allowed herself the indulgence of a cool, creamy, coffee-flavored drink* made with skim milk and sold at the same store. Clearly, she considered the low-fat drink to be much less of a high-carb crime than the chocolate-glazed cruller she longed for.

Ianna reported that as the weeks passed, her weight loss slowed to a halt. Although she had lost over twenty pounds on her low-carb diet prior to starting her new job, and had done it without cravings or struggle, each day now became a battle. Not only was she hungry "all of the time" but she had nothing in the way of weight loss to make it worth her while. In fact, she confessed, she had started to gain weight, though only a few pounds.

"It's just not worth it," she told us, adding that she didn't think she could hold on much longer.

We were faced with the unpleasant task of explaining Carb-Myth #2 to her and revealing that her cool, creamy coffee drink was not only laden with hidden carbs, it was clearly higher in carbohydrates than the food she had resisted so well. Ianna

---

*While we've used this example to illustrate the point that the carb counts of many foods may surprise you, it is only one of many examples you may find in a wide variety of products from many food manufacturers.

could have had a cruller—sugar, glazed, or topped with chocolate (her fantasy treat!)—and she would still have taken in fewer carbs and half the sugar of her skim milk coffee drink!

No wonder she wasn't losing weight. Her insulin levels were spiking during the entire time she stretched out the enjoyment of the drink, while her coworkers wolfed down their donuts in a matter of seconds. A double whammy: more carbs + a longer period of eating time = a longer time for insulin to keep socking away energy into the fat cells.

Ianna took the news well, which surprised and delighted us. "At least I know what's doing it," she explained. "And I'll have what I really want when I can have it."

Then she turned and added a final thought. "Imagine," she said, "if I hadn't had the skim milk variety. You know they also make it with cream instead."

We didn't want to tell her, but tell her we did. The cream version of her cold coffee drink was actually one gram lower in carbs and five grams lower in sugar.* Unwilling to believe it, she promised to show us that we were wrong when we saw her the following week, but seven days later, she returned with an acknowledgment that we were, indeed, correct. She'd read labels "like a hawk," she explained, and the results were clear.

Soon Ianna's cravings were gone. She lost two pounds in that first week and, with them, her fear that she would gain back all of the weight she'd fought so hard to lose.

Carb-Myth #3:
If I Don't Know What's in It, It Can't Hurt Me

This is one approach to dieting that, at some time or another, almost all of us succumb to. Richard and I sometimes refer to it as

---

*While we've used this example to illustrate the point that the carb counts of many foods may surprise you, it is only one of many examples you may find in a wide variety of products from many food manufacturers.

the Ostrich Approach to weight control. The Ostrich Approach is based on the belief that virtually any food that isn't obviously high-carb and has no label to prove otherwise can be considered low-carb.

> "After all, I can't fight the world. And, besides, how much damage can it do?"

Descent into the Ostrich Approach is usually marked by an unspoken gesture of surrender. A shrug and a smile of acceptance in response to a coworker's offer of a homemade dish that might, upon further examination, reveal a wide array of high-carb ingredients. Or the roll of your eyes at the back of the waiter who you know will never get your order as requested. Both confirm that although you know you are about to "fudge" on your diet, you have resigned yourself to giving up control.

"After all," you may tell yourself, "I can't fight the world. And, besides, how much damage can it do?"

This argument is similar to the one Richard and I hear from friends who are considering taking their kids out of school to go to Disney World. After all, they say, three days out of school isn't going to keep them from going to college, is it? The answer is a resounding "Could be!"

If their children are in second grade and they will be missing the last few days of school before summer vacation, it will probably do no harm. If, on the other hand, the youngsters are juniors in high school and are preparing for the college entrance exams or end-of-year finals, it might.

In the same way, giving in to the idea that "If I don't know what's in this food, it can't hurt me" can mean a great deal or not very much at all. The point is, you never know!

In our experience, low-carb dieters who eat food that they are not certain is truly low in carbohydrates are starting a downward descent that ends up with overwhelming cravings and weight-loss plateaus. When the party is over, or the special goodies are gone, or you've returned home from the restaurant, you may find yourself unable or unwilling to go back on your low-carb program. Or doing it halfheartedly, at best.

If, on the other hand, you find yourself right back on track as soon as you're back in your own territory, the weight-loss slow-down (or weight gain) that hits a day or two later may wipe away your motivation.

In either case, you may not realize that that "little slip" on your part has set the stage for going off your low-carb eating program. Letting things slide at restaurants, parties, or when dining at other people's homes can be the first step in a greater picture of not taking care of yourself.

Of most importance is *why* you're choosing to look the other way, neither questioning nor requesting the foods you need, not preparing or bringing with you food that is essential for your success. You'd do at least as much for a child, friend, family member, or even a pet who could not eat certain foods. You deserve at least as much consideration.

> Here is the best part;
> the greatest gift of all . . .

Each time you ask to see a label, request that a friend offer certain foods when you come for dinner, or request that a waiter bring you the food you need when you need it and prepared as you asked (without the side orders that simply *beg* to be nibbled on), each time you stand up for yourself and the goal you want, it becomes easier. You think about it less and feel more sure that you have a right to get what you need.

As you continue to take care of yourself, you will begin to respect how important your eating program and your weight loss are to you. That final piece of self-esteem—confidence in your right to get what you need in order to reach for your dreams—is one of the greatest gifts of all.

Confessions of an Ostrich: Simon's Story

About the same time that Ianna was coming to see us, we started a new round of research groups that included a young father who was determined to lose weight and keep it off in order to enjoy a long, healthy life with his wife and new son.

Like Ianna, Simon was the designated food fetcher. Although hired as a manager-in-training, his unwritten job description included a morning stop for his boss's breakfast at the local outlet of a well-known coffee franchise.*

Simon had lost quite a bit of weight on his low-carb program and had moved into a phase in which he allowed himself a limited amount of carbs each day.

Not wanting to "spend" all of his carbs on breakfast, Simon reported, he had avoided buying a bottle or two of the cold, creamy coffee drink* that tempted him and, instead, bought a "healthy" blueberry bagel at the bakery down the street.

"Everything at the bakery is homemade from scratch. I'm being *berry* good," he added, half apologizing for the pun. "I checked out the label on the drink* and it was almost twice what I ate in carbs all day when I started this diet.

"It's just not worth it," Simon added thoughtfully. "I worked too hard to take these forty-three pounds off to give it up for a three-minute drink."

When we asked how his morning bagel compared in carb count to the drink he was giving up, Simon looked surprised. He didn't know, he confessed, but "it's only a bagel with some berries thrown in and I'm allowed to have berries now. Besides, all I put on it is cream cheese."

Rather than argue the point, we asked him if he'd mind

---

*While we've used this example to illustrate the point that the carb counts of many foods may surprise you, it is only one of many examples you may find in a wide variety of products from many food manufacturers.

doing a bit of detective work. Although he confessed to feeling a little uneasy about asking the bakery woman for more information on the bagels, for fear of insulting her, we pushed the issue and he agreed.

The following week, Simon had some news to share.

"I did it. I didn't want to, but I did," he began. He handed us an empty plastic bag, and we read the nutritional label.

Simon's "treat" contained sixty-nine carbs.
With the insulin spike that was sure to
follow, no wonder he was starving by 11 A.M.

By asking for more information, Simon had discovered two things: First, that his blueberry bagel contained sixty-nine carbs, almost twice that of the bottled drink he had considered too high in carbs to have for breakfast. Second, that his "homemade" bagel came frozen to the bakery, which was, in fact, one of several stores in a larger franchise.

"All they were doing was warming it up in a microwave," Simon said, shaking his head. "And sixty-nine carbs at that! No wonder I've been starving every day by eleven A.M."

His powerful breakthrough brought Simon
and his family a wonderful new life.

"Well, you've learned two valuable lessons," we offered, hoping to show him the positive side of the experience.

"Three," Simon corrected. "This weekend I took my son to the zoo. Standing there, looking at the ostriches, I kept wishing they'd put their heads in the sand so my son could see. Then I realized that that's what I've been doing, not just with the bagel but with other things that I've been eating. And it's why I've stopped weighing myself altogether."

With that final revelation, Simon made a breakthrough to success that has grown along with his young son (and second son, as well). Just as he had been hiding from the facts of what his food contained, he was avoiding truths about changes in his eating, his weight, and his willingness to look reality in the face and make it work for him.

As a result of being more honest with himself, Simon made far better breakfast choices, his mid-morning cravings disappeared, and he enjoyed an easy success in both his diet and his weight loss. He confessed that his willingness to confront the unknown improved his marriage as well. (Although he smiled warmly when he told us, he never offered any details.)

We, on the other hand, chose to be a little less than frank with Simon, at least for the moment. We never told him that while the ostrich may lower its head to escape detection by predators or use its bill to dig a shallow nest, the idea that it sticks its head in the sand is pure myth.

The way we figure it, there's no need to weigh Simon down with unnecessary facts. Our bird is flying high!

Carb-Myth #4:

If It's Good for You, It Can't Be So Bad

This myth comes in several variations:

If it's good for you, it can't be so bad for your diet.
If it's healthy, it can't be so bad for your diet.
If it's natural, it can't be so bad for your diet.
If you only have a little bit, it can't be so bad for your diet.

All of the above variations have one thing in common: when it comes to following a low-carb program, they are all definitely, decidedly, and totally untrue.

In the world of sales, especially when it comes to food, image is everything. If food manufacturers can get you to see one food as "healthy" and another as "bad for you," the images that surround those foods will influence your choice even in the face of facts that clearly disprove them.

Some images are self-perpetuating; certain foods "look" like they should be healthful. Other images take a bit more persuasion. In the past, convenience, low-cost, and practicality were big selling points. When margarine first hit the market, for instance, it had a big low-cost element going for it (though it lacked convenience because you had to mix in the yellow coloring that made it look more appealing).*

> The ingredients in foods may change
> but once we think of a food as "good
> for us" the image tends to stick.

Food image today is driven, almost without exception, by a blatant appeal to healthfulness (or rather the avoidance or reversal of risk for illness). Packaged products of every kind offer hope of reduced cholesterol levels, decreased risk of heart attack, or the like. Taken to the extreme, if we're to believe all that we're told, we could convince ourselves that if we just ate enough of the right things, we could live forever.

Even when the food of today barely resembles the product that originally earned the sterling reputation, we still tend to see it as a "healthy" food. It is equally difficult for a food or drink that has been categorized as "fattening" to lose that reputation.

> Ounce for ounce, which is higher
> in carbs: beer or vegetable juice?

---

*While we've used this example to illustrate our point, it is only one of many examples you may find in a wide variety of products from many food manufacturers.

Here's a question to tap your knowledge of carb counts. Ounce for ounce, which is higher in carbs: beer or vegetable juice?

The answer: The average eight-ounce glass of beer contains four carbs, as compared with ten carbs in the same amount of vegetable juice (most of which is sugar).*

This example is clearly not meant to indicate that beer is a better choice than vegetable juice, which may legitimately claim any of a variety of health-improving benefits. But it's essential to your success to remember that while one food may carry an image of healthfulness and the other may not, their carb counts may be quite separate and distinct from these images.

Help At Your Fingertips

Even if you knew the answer to the beer vs. vegetable question above, we don't want you to get too sure of yourself! Knowing how to spot hidden carbohydrates is so important that even old veterans like us have to depend on some help.

Your low-carb plan may require you to count carbs, or you may use a list of foods as a guide when making your low-carb choices. In any case, if you're on any kind of a low-carb diet, a carbohydrate counter can be an essential tool.

> A good carb counter can
> buy you more pleasure.

Though you may never count carbs, a quick look at a carb counter can tell you which choices will give you the most pleasure for your carb spending. You may discover that the food you are really craving (and that you thought was too high in

---

*While we've used this example to illustrate the point that the carb counts of many foods may surprise you, it is only one of many examples you may find in a wide variety of products from many food manufacturers.

carbs) is actually quite acceptable. Or you might discover that by choosing a different dressing on your salad you can also have that bit of dessert you've been dreaming about.

Choose any counter you feel you can rely on. Make sure it's easy to read (especially for quick reference) and detailed enough to give you the information you need. Most important, make certain it uses standard measurement. It's almost impossible, for instance, to compare a half cup of one vegetable with four ounces by weight of another. So be certain your counter uses the same weight, measurement, or serving within a category.

Here's an example from one carbohydrate counter we think works well. It's our own book, *The Carbohydrate Addict's Carbohydrate Counter,* and it illustrates what a carbohydrate counter should do.

For a moment, imagine that you are about to eat out at a deli, and while you are allowed some carbohydrates on your plan, you aren't sure how things stack up in comparison. You are not about to sit there and figure the carb count for each slice of bread, piece of meat, and condiment that makes up each sandwich. Nor do you want to have to search through the counter to find the carb counts of typical side dishes.

Using our *Carbohydrate Addict's Carbohydrate Counter* or any other counter that offers you similar information at your fingertips, you can make informed choices, then sit back and enjoy your meal.

Dining Out: DELICATESSEN*

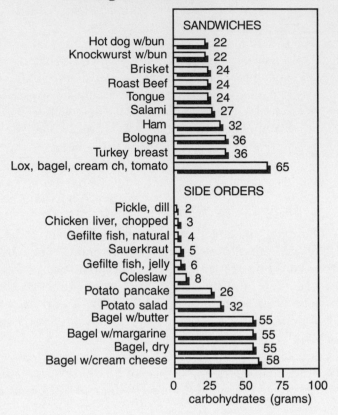

*Unless otherwise indicated, counts based on average-size servings or sandwiches. Sandwich counts assume white or rye bread.

Chapter 14

TAMING THE HUNGER HORMONE

If It Ain't Broke, Still Fix It!

Most people live by the rule that says "If it ain't broke, don't fix it." These are the same people who will ignore the rattle in the car, the blurriness on the TV screen, and the warning signs that they are about to go off their low-carb diet. Unwilling to trust the fact that things don't get better by themselves, but rather almost certainly get worse, they look the other way and wait for the car or TV to stop working completely, or for their eating and weight to get so out of control that they're tempted to give up completely.

> You can pull yourself back onto your program
> before you ever really go off.

We have a completely different point of view and one that we have found almost certainly leads to success and a feeling of control over one's weight and life. By being aware of the five Warning Signs that indicate you are about to go off your low-carb eating plan, you can stop the problem before it gets out of hand and pull yourself back onto your program before you ever really go off.

As any low-carb dieter will tell you, it's easier to *stay* on your program than to climb back on. If you have fallen off, go to Day #1 of the 7-Day Jump-Start Plan and, day by day, bring your body back into balance so that you can move back into your low-carb program most easily.

Once you have made it back onto your program, or if you are still on it but faltering or struggling, knowing and acting on the Warning Signs you'll find in this chapter can help keep you right on track.

> Chances are you're used to ignoring your
> own discomforts, needs, and desires.

Our job is to tell you what signs to look out for and what to do about them. Your job, on the other hand, is to take action when the Warning Signs occur. If you typically ignore your own discomforts, needs, and desires—all messages that your body "wants" something—you need to pay attention. When it comes to Warning Signs, you must take them as seriously as you would a rash that comes from eating a food that you are allergic to or the backache that says you've been lifting too many heavy things. Both are telling you to stop, look, and listen to your body. If you don't, problems are almost sure to follow.

> You'll find Rescue (immediate and concrete
> help to get you out of the situation fast) and
> Recovery (long-term help and prevention).

In these pages, you'll find many of the Warning Signs that can mean your insulin levels are out of balance and that a struggle with your eating or a fall off the low-carb wagon is about to occur. After each Warning Sign, you'll find Rescue—immediate and concrete help to get you out of the situation fast—and Recovery—

long-term help and prevention. In most cases, we'll tell you what you should do *right away*, and depending on the problem, we'll either offer you some recommendations for avoiding the problem in the future or, rather than repeat ourselves, point you to another section of this book for further help.

We have found (the hard way) that Warning Signs are precious gifts that should not be ignored. They can help you succeed only if you pay attention to them.

Both of us remember one young man who came to us because he experienced recurring signs of hypoglycemia (low blood sugar) that always showed up within an hour or two after eating. Testing showed that the sweats, confusion, and weakness he experienced were his body's way of saying that although he thought he was eating low-carb foods, some high-carb foods were still getting into his system. He had been ignoring these symptoms for months until, by the time he came to us, he had accepted them as part of his life and begun to reorganize his life around them.

As a surgeon, he was careful to schedule his procedures for the early morning and did not eat until the last patient had been taken care of. He put his afternoon rounds on hold until three hours after lunch, allowing him time to pull out of the low blood sugar reaction that was almost sure to follow his meal. The rest of the day he experienced a series of blood sugar ups and downs. Since he thought he was following a low-carb diet, on top of all the other difficulties, he didn't understand why he wasn't losing any weight.

After intense instruction on the importance of attending to his Warning Signs (we yelled at him!), our young surgeon took action at the first sign of a low blood sugar swing. Having a supply of assuredly low-carb food available (rather than the sugar-laden candies he had been resorting to), he was able to pull out of the low blood sugar swing without insulin rebound. Going to work immediately to find the source of the problem, he discovered that the hospital cafeteria at which he had been getting his meals had been serving him tuna salad laced with fillers, scrambled eggs loaded with glutamates, and sausages filled with both. No matter what he ate, his insulin surged and his blood sugar crashed. Had he been diabetic and his blood sugar had risen, he would have made the connection, but he had shrugged off the low blood sugar reaction, attributing it to his "being on a diet" or "just not getting enough food."

A new cafeteria, and the low blood
sugar swings were gone, along with
more than twenty pounds.

A simple change in cafeterias, from the main dining room to the upstairs lunchroom that catered to hospital personnel who required fewer "processed" foods, changed the whole experience of his day and his diet. The hypoglycemia disappeared and, over the next few months, so did more than twenty pounds.

In the same way, understanding and paying attention to the Warning Signs that follow can help you Rescue your low-carb program and Recover your ability to achieve the changes you'd like to make real.

IMPORTANT NOTICE BEFORE YOU BEGIN: Each of the Warning Signs that follow can indicate serious physical problems that should be attended to by a health care professional. Before using our Rescue and Recovery suggestions, see your physician and make absolutely certain that no physical problem or disorder is causing or contributing to your symptoms. In addition, be certain to get your physician's okay before taking any Rescue action that may not be in keeping with your personal health concerns or requirements.

Sweating, confusion, and/or weakness
within an hour or two after eating

Warning Sign #1:

Sweating, Confusion, and/or Weakness within an hour or two after eating

These clearly physical symptoms are often signs that you are experiencing a low blood sugar swing in response to a surge of insulin, probably as a result of consuming hidden carbohydrates or Carbohydrate Act-Alikes (such as glutamates and/or sugar substitutes) in your food or drink.

Rescue: Immediately eat some low-carb protein that you are certain does not contain any hidden carbohydrates or Carbohydrate Act-Alikes. Several pieces of cheese (cheddar or Swiss seem to work well) or some home-cooked meat, fish, or fowl should do. Canned tuna is easy to keep on hand, but be certain it is the low-salt variety that does not contain any glutamates under the ingredient names broth, hydrolyzed soy protein, hydrolyzed food protein, natural flavors, or the like.* Chew the food well (though you may be tempted to wolf it down) and drink some plain cool water with it. If you don't feel relief within only a few minutes, repeat the low-protein snack with water.

Recovery: Do not repeatedly rely on the Rescue strategy above to bring your blood sugar levels back into balance. After making certain there is no underlying medical problem, it is essential that you find the source of the hidden carbohydrates or Carbohydrate Act-Alikes. Read Chapters 12 and 13 in this book, which deal with these topics.

If you knowingly ate high-carbohydrate foods or drinks that contained sugar substitutes, you need to seriously consider whether you want to keep putting your body through such an ordeal and suffering the possible health consequences. Not everyone reacts to high-carb foods and/or sugar substitutes and glutamates in the same way, but if you react strongly and negatively, it's a really bad idea to continue to ignore their presence in your food. If you're having trouble getting yourself to make a change,

---

*For more information on glutamates, see the chapter "Five Vital Clues Low-Carb Diet Doctors Miss."

see our chapters "Healthy Selfishness" and "Five Vital Clues Low-Carb Diet Doctors Miss." In addition, it's always a good idea to seek the support and motivation you need from a health care professional or counselor so that you can be more certain of taking good care of yourself.

> Intense or recurring cravings especially for
> starches, snack foods, junk food, or sweets

Warning Sign #2:

Intense or Recurring Cravings, especially for starches, snack foods, junk food, or sweets

These can be signs that you are experiencing a surge in insulin or prolonged high levels of insulin, which may come from eating high-carb foods frequently (or in great amounts) or from consuming hidden carbohydrates or Carbohydrate Act-Alikes (such as glutamates and/or sugar substitutes) in your food or drink.

Rescue: Get away from all immediate sources of food and drink. Don't tell yourself you can handle it . . . *get outta there, now.* If you need to, go to the bathroom so that you can get some time to think rationally and plan how to get through the next hour or so without going off your program (or going off it even more than you may already have).

If you are in a carbo spiral (that is, you eat something high-carb, tell yourself you won't do it again, then find yourself eating more high-carbs a couple of hours later—or sooner), get out of the situation as quickly as humanly possible.

Whether you are in a carbo spiral or not, eat some low-carb protein (such as the cheese, meat, fish, and/or fowl we describe in Warning Sign #1). Make certain the protein is free of hidden carbohydrates and Carbohydrate Act-Alikes. Chew it well and be sure to drink some cool water with it.

If, and only if, you are certain you can control your eating in spite of the cravings, you can go back to the environment where your cravings first hit. Don't go back to a situation you can't handle, especially one that combines available food with no time to think (such as a party or business meeting). If the cravings return, get out of the situation until you can better prepare for it with the Recovery recommendations that follow.

Recovery: There are only so many times you can make a mad dash for the bathroom in response to intense urges to eat, without drawing attention to yourself. On the other hand, most people become so used to feeling cravings that they stop thinking there's anything unusual about them and assume that everyone has intense and driving cravings for high-carb food, which is decidedly not true.

Cravings are one of the most disregarded and helpful Warning Signs. Unfortunately, few people give them the credit they deserve. When reporters and television interviewers ask us for our best-kept secrets and tips on successful weight loss, we always put paying attention to telltale cravings at the top of our list. Cravings can tell you where the hidden carbs and Carbohydrate Act-Alikes are concealed—usually in the food or drink that you consumed only one to two hours earlier.

When it comes to cravings, it's essential to neither shrug them off nor explain them away. Find the source of the hidden carbohydrates or Carbohydrate Act-Alikes in your food.

Intentionally eating high-carb foods frequently or in great amounts, or consuming drinks that contain sugar substitutes, can produce surprisingly intense cravings, in particular for starches, snack foods, junk foods, or sweets. If you're having trouble getting off the carbo spiral, go to the Day #1 chapter of this book and begin moving through the 7-Day Jump-Start Plan. At the same time, read through the rest of this book to learn about the unexpected triggers that might be throwing you off track. Enlist a friend's help or get the support and motivation you need from a health care professional or counselor. Going off your eating program starts long before you put the first bite of a "trigger food" in your mouth. Get rid of the hidden carbs, Carbohydrate Act-Alikes, and the frequent or excessive intake of high-carb foods, and you'll probably see the cravings vanish as well.

> Headache or irritability or a profound
> tiredness either immediately or within two
> hours after eating

Warning Signs #3, #4, And #5:

Headache, Irritability, or a Profound Tiredness either immediately or within two hours after eating

These can be typical signs of high insulin levels causing the shutdown of cells to their source of nourishment (that is, blood sugar). Just as blood sugar levels can drop too quickly for some, in others who may be more insulin resistant,* high levels of this hunger- and fat-making hormone can shut down the cells' ability to take in sugar.

While your cells starve for much-needed nutrition, you may feel a cascade of physical reactions that include headache and irritability (as the nervous system strains to get the energy it needs) or excessive or profound tiredness (as muscle cells are robbed of their nutrition). Blood sugar may be trapped in the bloodstream along with the high levels of insulin, setting the stage for adult-onset diabetes.

Rescue: Ongoing post-meal headaches, irritability, or a profound sense of tiredness must be taken very seriously. While an immediate Rescue tactic is the same as that used in Warning Sign #1, we strongly recommend that you go immediately to Recovery and eliminate the cause of this more advanced problem.

Recovery: Ongoing post-meal headaches, irritability, or profound tiredness can be signs of an ongoing insulin problem, including but not limited to insulin resistance. We believe they require evaluation by a physician. While it appears that the con-

---

*That is, a condition in which your body is no longer able to handle frequent or intense surges of insulin and reduces the number of places (or sites) through which cells can get needed fuel. You can find a more in-depth explanation and discussion of insulin resistance in our book *Healthy for Life*.

sumption of high-carb foods frequently or in inappropriate quantities, or the intake of hidden carbohydrates or Carbohydrate Act-Alikes, may play a significant role in causing, worsening, or exacerbating insulin resistance, this medical problem should be ruled out or treated by your physician.

Chapter 15

TROUBLESHOOTING

If The Car's Out Of Gas . . . Don't Dump It!

Imagine that a friend calls, and in the course of the conversation, you learn that she bought a car recently, and it worked pretty well, was comfortable, dependable, and took her where she wanted to go. But while she was driving along that morning, the car stopped running . . . so she coasted over to the side of the road and walked away.

You might ask how she plans to get it going again. She then informs you that she has no intention of doing anything about it. She's had many cars in the past, some of which ran well and others that had problems from the start. Yet, in every case, as each car stopped running, she would abandon it, going carless for a while until her next automobile purchase . . . with the same ultimate result.

You might assume your friend is joking or, at the very least, being amazingly foolish. You might try and explain that her car might have developed only a minor problem, something that could be easily fixed by someone who knew how to diagnose and correct the problem. Why, the car might only have run out of gas! You find your friend is not listening.

Giving up, you say goodbye and return to your own thoughts. Now, where were you? Oh, yes, you had just decided to give up on your low-carb diet; it worked well for a while but lately you've been struggling to stay on it and find that you're barely losing any weight at all.

"Well, that's that!" you conclude. "They're all the same in the end."

This scenario is just our way of making the point, if the car's out of gas . . . don't dump the car!

Whether you are hitting a few bumps on the road or facing a virtual obstacle course of low-carb diet challenges, you may find that the TroubleShooting help within the pages of this chapter is all you need to get back on track.

A Quick Course In Success

Problem

Whenever I start to cheat on a diet, low-carb or otherwise, I know it's the beginning of the end. I might struggle for a while, but eventually, I know I'm going to fail. With me, either I do it perfectly or not at all.

> Once I start to cheat, it's all over.

TroubleShooter

That's it, that's exactly the thinking we want you to hear . . . and help you get rid of! When it comes to dieting, people seem to take an "all or nothing" stance. Most of us are so afraid of failing yet again that we find it easier and less disheartening to give up than to fix each problem as it appears.

We all know that a toddler learns to walk by trying, falling, figuring out what went wrong, and trying again. He repeats the process over and over again until soon he's dashing around without a worry in the world. If he had given up on the first try, or the twentieth, he'd still be sitting in the corner.

Most of us have come to accept that in certain areas of our

lives, trial and error is the acceptable—in fact, the only—way to learn. Unfortunately, most dieters don't consider trial and error acceptable.

> Most of us are encyclopedias on
> how *not* to succeed on a diet.

If you are a diet perfectionist, a hard-on-yourself do-it-right-or-not-at-all tyrant, give yourself a break. Success is learned, either through your own attempts (and failures) or by observing others. It took Thomas Edison nearly eight thousand "failures" before he found a material that would produce a light bulb. When asked what he had learned from the experience, he simply said that he now knew of seven thousand and ninety-nine materials that could not be used to make a light bulb. Most of us know many, many ways *not* to succeed on a diet. Success comes simply by putting this vast knowledge to work for you.

As you read the pages that follow (and the other chapters of the book), we urge you to confront your diet roadblocks, one by one, with the same conviction with which you would tackle any problem that a friend or family member might have.

Make sure that any program you choose works for you, is one that your doctor approves of, and one that you can maintain for life.

No matter which program you choose, focus on any problems you may be encountering as rationally as possible, one at a time, just like Thomas Edison did for the light bulb. Find the TroubleShooting tip that addresses your concern. Then work out a plan to handle that problem—a solution that's right for *you*—and do it!

In life, as in dieting, there is only one real failure—the failure to learn from your mistakes. So long as you are learning, you have not failed. After all, each of us is only "a work in progress."

Your job is simply this: to keep learning, to get better and better at reaching toward your goal, to stop judging, and to not give up.

Willpower Hijackers

Problem

I get incredible cravings for high-carb foods. Sometimes I simply have no will power.

When your craving for carbs
is overwhelming . . .

TroubleShooter

Sometimes people think that even more than chocolate, a lack of willpower keeps them overweight.

Wrong! When a little lab rat is given a treatment that throws his insulin levels out of balance, he will begin to gorge himself on carbohydrate-rich chow. The poor little lab rat hasn't suddenly lost his willpower; his body is driving him to the food. When humans have too much insulin in their blood, the same thing happens. It's not a matter of willpower; it's a matter of biology.

You have probably seen the proof yourself. Chances are there have been times when, no matter what you did, you couldn't get enough food . . . in particular, starches, snack foods, junk food, and sweets. We bet you've never heard of anyone binging on celery. There have probably been other times when you couldn't have cared less about food or, at least, when you had no trouble controlling what you ate.

The reason for the great difference in your feelings—in your need—for food was not willpower but, more likely, changes in your body chemistry that were stimulating your need for high-carb foods.

High-carb foods cause insulin surges, which, in turn, call for more high-carb foods. The more *often* you have them, the more often you want them. And the more of them you eat, the more of them you crave. Other factors, like monthly hormonal changes, stress, boredom, loneliness, the simple act of aging, certain medications, additives in your food, lack of sleep, and anxiety can all trigger intense and recurring cravings for high-carb foods.

The first place to look for the *cause* of intense cravings for high-carb foods is in the last food you ate. In most cases, you'll find hidden carbohydrates in food that you thought or were told was low-carb.

What worries us most these days is the many processed foods that imply or claim that they're low-carb while containing ingredients that are *known* to cause insulin surges. Performing all sorts of mathematical computations, food manufacturers come up with numbers that make their "low-carb" candy bars, shakes, and desserts look like they will help you lose weight.

Although most dieters know in their hearts that a "low-carb creamy chocolate cheesecake" and a "low-carb strawberry shake" are just too good to be true, they never connect these forays into low-carb fantasy with the cravings they get two or three hours later.

If you are getting cravings for high-carb foods or if you find yourself "cheating," we strongly suggest that you make sure you're eating real food that's genuinely low-carb (meat, chicken, fish, and low-carb vegetables), not something that came "prepared." You're almost certain to see your cravings disappear.

Don't be tempted to conclude that low-carb diets don't work when, without your knowledge, you haven't really been on one.

Learn which foods contain hidden carbohydrates and watch out for Carbohydrate Act-Alikes such as sugar substitutes, glutamates, and saturated fats. The cravings that follow can challenge even the strongest resolve.

Most importantly, when the cravings hit, don't blame yourself. It's an old habit that isn't warranted and doesn't work. Do something different! Look at what you've been eating and drinking (either within the last two hours or throughout the day). When you find the culprit that's been "stealing" your so-called willpower, you'll know who's really to blame.

Low-Carb Smart: Quick Meals, Please

Problem

I don't have time to make low-carb meals. And, quite honestly, it's just too much trouble. Besides, I get bored with the same old food, day after day. I dare you to fix that!

> Your low-carb meals can be
> fun and exciting. Really!

TroubleShooter

You bet! First, if you are thinking that going low-carb takes time or trouble, you aren't thinking low-carb smart! Consider our own Great American Cookout (actually more like a Cook-In). Once a week, we go shopping for every low-carb food we can think of. Heading back to the kitchen, we put on our favorite movie (from our collection or rented for this very purpose) and start cookin' like crazy.

While a couple of chickens are baking in the oven, we cut up vegetables to be stir-fried and frozen in meal-size portions. If money is a real concern, buy whichever protein is on sale so long as you'll enjoy it; turkey is usually a great buy and one big bird can make a whole lot of low-carb meals.

Most salad makings can be prepared at the same time and stored away for the next three days. Dips and dressings can be made in advance and frozen for later use. When the chickens are done, we throw some steaks or chops in the broiler, to be eaten that night, the leftovers to be mixed with the stir-fried vegetables.

When the chicken is fully cooled, we take off the wings and legs, then cut slices of the meat and freeze them in the gravy. The bits that remain make perfect pieces to be combined with celery in a low-carb chicken salad.

Within a couple of hours, we've made lunches and dinners for the week and some extra breakfast goodies as well. We've spent less time (and money) than if we weren't on a diet at all, or had prepared each meal separately, and it was a lot of fun! Even better, we have minimized the impact of food additives that are so rampant in prepared and processed foods.

Low-Carb boredom has to be treated as a serious threat to your weight-loss success. You've got to keep a good variety in your daily meals. To keep things interesting, we try to serve two or more proteins and two vegetable dishes at every lunch and dinner. We freeze half-size servings and take out two different kinds at a time. Or, if we're cooking that night, we make extra for the next night, to ensure that we've got a good supply of leftovers.

We like chicken and meat (pork or beef) in the same meal but prefer fish only with other seafood like shrimp and scallops. That's just our preference; yours may be different. In any case, don't restrict yourself to one protein or one vegetable. You'll get real bored, real fast. No variety? That's simply no fun! And adding variety to your diet doesn't have to take a chunk of time or money out of your day. With a little ingenuity you can have a buffet at every meal.

Have a Great American Cookout of your own. Just pretend you've got family (a very big family) coming over for dinner. Then package up all the food and keep it for yourself!

Getting Things Moving Again: Constipation

Problem

When I eat low-carb, I get constipated—badly! What do you do?

Constipated? We have an answer
that's amazingly effective.

TroubleShooter

First, it's essential to make certain that your constipation is not due to some medical condition. Don't automatically assume it comes from eating low-carb; check it out with your physician and be sure. Certain medical problems, lack of exercise, and medications are only some of the many factors that can lead to constipation.

Once your doctor determines that the only cause of your constipation is your low-carb diet, ask him/her if it's okay to try the "amazingly effective method" that works so well for us. We laugh about it because it's absurdly simple.

No artificial ingredients, no bottles to buy, no pills to take . . . just eat two large stalks of celery every day, preferably at the same meal or snack. It's a good idea to drink a large glass of water with it, but we don't know if that's necessary. That's it! The amazingly effective method that has kept us constipation free!

No other vegetable works half as well for us, and as dozens of waiters will tell you, we order it even when we're on the road. It takes a second to explain to the waiter that you want "a side order of plain, raw celery." Your waiter may hesitate at first and tell you that he's not sure the chef can prepare it for you. We explain that we need it for "medical reasons" or "for our health" and we almost always get it.

Lately, we've been ordering celery immediately upon sitting down at the table, at the same time we order our iced teas. We ask them to bring it as soon as possible and get to crunch and munch on the celery while we're waiting for our first course. In that way if it's one of our low-carb meals, we have something to eat in place of bread, or if it's our Reward Meal,* chewing on the celery helps us hold on until we've finished our lower-carb food and it's time to enjoy our starches and dessert. In either case it's a win-win for staying on our diet and helping to eliminate constipation—sort of killing two problems with one celery stalk (actually two).

---

*For more information on Reward Meals and including high-carb foods in one meal each day, see our *Carbohydrate Addict's LifeSpan Program* book.

Make certain that you're drinking enough water. When you are eating foods low in carbohydrates and your cravings diminish or disappear, you may be less likely to drink the fluids you need. Also, as you naturally start to snack less often, you will—once again—be drinking less. In addition, since insulin signals your body to retain salt and salt signals your body to retain fluid, as your insulin levels decrease, you will most likely tend to retain less fluid.

In order to have normal, regular bowel movements, your body needs a sufficient amount of liquid, so to make up for your tendency to drink less and your body's tendency to retain less liquid when you are eating low-carb, you'll have to make a concerted effort to drink more (preferably, good old water). The quantity of liquid you should be taking in each day is best determined by your physician. Age, weight, build, lifestyle, medication and health concerns can all influence the right amount for you.

Cracking The Breakfast Dilemma

Problem

I am tired of eggs for breakfast, and I don't want to eat one of those "low-carb meal replacement bars." I can't stop with just one and they always leave me hungry before lunch. What can I eat for low-carb breakfasts?

> If I have to eat one more egg for breakfast, I'll cluck!

TroubleShooter

There is absolutely no need to eat eggs every day for breakfast. You are probably resorting to them as the only way out of your Breakfast Dilemma. Like you, others have discovered that "low-carb meal replacement bars"* do more to stimulate their appetite than satisfy it, leaving them wanting more and more (and often eating more and more as well).

Breakfast Dilemmas are solved easily with a change in thinking. First, if you possibly can, challenge the rule that says breakfast food should be different than the food served at other meals. The switch to high-carb breakfasts in this country came during World War II when protein was being shipped to our soldiers. Propaganda messages popped up everywhere, extolling the pleasures and benefits of cold cereals and breakfasts composed almost entirely of high-carb foods.

The American public ate it up (literally and figuratively!). Within a short time, the usual three or four brands of cold cereal had grown to dozens. Now supermarkets boast over two hundred kinds of cereal, almost all of which contain sugar. With more women trying to meet the demands of work and family, cereals, breads, and baked goods became the breakfast norm. Pop them into the toaster, eat them cold, eat them on the run— you name it. The low-fat phase of dieting sounded the final death knell to a protein-rich breakfast in the U.S., although bangers (sausage) and kippers (fish) are still served for breakfast in England, as are similar low-carb protein choices around the world.

So the first way out of the Breakfast Dilemma is to open your mind to new (and old) choices. Consider all of the low-carb foods that you might enjoy for breakfast, including those you might have at a buffet (such as poached salmon, shrimp, sliced turkey or chicken). Have them ready and fresh for the taking. Certainly, one can rely on celery stuffed with cream cheese for only so long. Our *Carbohydrate Addict's Cookbook* offers twenty-five low-carb breakfast recipes (from Breakfast Pockets to Hearty Breakfast Quiche and beyond) and dozens of appetizers, quick fix dishes, and snacks to wake up your breakfasts and remind you that food is meant to be enjoyed.

---

*For more information on "low carb" processed foods and cravings and weight-loss slowdown, see "Willpower Hijackers" in this chapter as well as the "Five Vital Clues Low-Carb Diet Doctors Miss" chapter in this book.

For some, however, almost nothing tastes good in the morning. They may be able to enjoy a bagel, toast, or cereal, but they are really not hungry in the morning and find themselves eating because they've been told it's good for them.

Certainly, we could argue the validity (or the lack of the validity) of studies that claim that *everyone* needs a good breakfast. In truth, since it takes many hours for our bodies to move the food out of our stomachs and through the digestive system where the nutrients are absorbed into the body, it's probably far more accurate to say that the food you eat in the morning fuels you during the night, and the food you eat at dinner fuels you through the next day.

In addition, we wonder about the vested interests that are trying to convince an entire nation that missing or postponing breakfast is not good for you. We have to admit that we think it would be more accurate to say it's not good for *them*.

Once again, you must check with your physician, but we believe that for most people who are trying to lose weight, to skip or postpone a meal because you aren't hungry is perfectly acceptable. When you're trying to lose weight, to eat when you are not hungry makes no sense at all.

So if your doctor agrees, when you don't want to eat breakfast, don't do it! Or, as so many people have found, it's fun to postpone it until mid-morning (around 11:00 A.M. or so). There are perfectly healthy people who eat two meals a day and others who find they only want one meal a day. Each of us is different. Chances are you'll have no difficulty including a whole array of low-carb foods in the meal that more resembles a lunch than a breakfast.

Among the people who have used this last solution to the Breakfast Dilemma, we've noticed two interesting patterns. By delaying breakfast until mid-morning, about half of them eventually forget about breakfast, and make lunch their first meal. The other half enjoy a satisfying low-carb brunch but forget to have the late lunch they had planned on. A few do manage to have both meals but report they are eating out of "habit" rather than hunger and, after a while, often choose to skip one meal or the other.

Remember not to *force* yourself to give up a meal. If you want it, have it. And if you decide you'd like to experiment and skip a meal or postpone it, that option is always yours. If there's no reason to push yourself to eat, low-carb or otherwise, why do it?

Generally, during the week, we don't have breakfast, just a cup of coffee or tea. We don't really want breakfast (but if we did, we would have it). An early lunch starts our eating day. And by then we're ready for it.

Weekends, for us, are a whole different matter. We sleep a bit later, and when we get up, we're ready for a good meal. That's when we enjoy the pleasures of a hot breakfast, and because we haven't been faced with the Breakfast Dilemma all week, we savor every minute and every mouthful of a wide variety of low-carb food, and if it's our Reward Meal, high-carb treats as well.

Vacations, Parties, And Holidays

Problem

I blew my low-carb diet on vacation. Big time!

I lost my diet over the holidays. It was impossible to stay on it.

I don't want to be the only one at the party nibbling on celery and watching while everyone else is eating everything in sight.

> Three low-carb diet assassins:
> parties, vacations, and holidays.

TroubleShooter

They're the top three killers of low-carb diets: parties, vacations, and holidays. They are fraught with minefields of temptation. And they are easy to handle, if you just know how.

The first question to ask yourself is "Is it *possible* to stay on my low-carb diet on this vacation, or at this party?" If you can answer yes only by planning to eat and drink nothing but water, you're not being realistic.

You can't be expected to go to a party, stand around all night, and eat nothing. Or to nibble on some wilted celery while continuing to resist the sights and smells that surround you. You may hold out for a little while, rewarding yourself with feelings of self-righteousness. You may even last the night. But sooner or later, this time or next, you're almost bound to give in and throw your low-carb program to the wind.

So, looking *realistically* at the situation, you need to decide if attending the event while sticking to your low-carb diet is doable. In many cases, to make certain you have the low-carb food you need, you'll have to bring it *yourself.*

"Friend failure" is a very common cause of diet breakdowns. Your friend or family member assures you that there will be lots of low-carb food for you to choose from at a party or dinner, but for one reason on another, they almost always fail to keep their promise.

"There are lots of people coming who are on that diet," they assure you. "We've been on it ourselves."

The last line should be a giveaway. If they did so well on the diet, they'd still be on it. And when you arrive, you find out why they failed. The low-carb food that was promised simply isn't there. Or it's covered in high-carb dressings or mixed in with high-carb foods. What your hosts consider "low-carb" is beyond your comprehension, and the other guests who were supposed to be bringing low-carb dishes didn't.

You are left high and dry in carb country. Is it any wonder you just give in? If you don't, you're one in a million; if you do, you're only human. Here's what will help.

Next time, make certain that your expectations are realistic. The only way to be certain of sticking to a low-carb eating plan at a party is to bring all the food you want to eat. Bring extras. There will be other low-carb dieters who will be desperate for help. If there's not enough to go around, put yourself first and, if you must, deny them the food that will keep you on your program. It may seem heartless and selfish, but sometimes it's a matter of survival.

Richard and I have had the experience of giving other guests some of our low-carb goodies, food we brought with us to parties or dinners. After sharing our limited supply (you can only bring so much), we watched the same guests who had eaten up our food polish off several high-carb treats. So much for bringing enough for the whole class.

So, when facing a party, decide if low-carb is doable and, if it is, bring the food you need. If, on the other hand, low-carb eating is clearly not a viable alternative, temporarily move to an eating program that will allow you some carbohydrates while helping to keep your insulin levels in balance. In particular, of course, we recommend our Carbohydrate Addict's LifeSpan Program because it allows for a balanced Reward Meal that includes high-carb foods. That way, you can enjoy the party and some high-carb treats, including an alcoholic drink or two, *in balance* and within the guidelines that will help protect you from an insulin rebound.

The next day, following the party, you can return to your low-carb program with less worry of weight gain or craving rebound. Or, if you like, you can remain with our program and enjoy the benefits of a daily Reward Meal while continuing to reap the weight-loss and craving-reducing benefits of a low-carb diet.

A special tactic that works well for parties and catered affairs such as weddings involves eating a hearty low-carb meal before you go. After you arrive, hold on the first hour or two before you enjoy a balanced Reward Meal. You might carry a plate on which you place the hors d'oeuvres you plan to eat a little later. You'll seem to be nibbling like everyone else. At two-meal affairs (an hors d'oeuvre hour followed by a sit-down dinner, for instance) choose one meal as a designated low-carb meal (the buffet is usually the best choice) and the other as a balanced Reward Meal.

Whether you go low-carb at the party or enjoy it as your Reward Meal, you must plan ahead; think it through as you would any task at which you want to succeed. As a starting point, use some of the strategies you will find in our chapter "Restaurant Tactics" and add to the wealth of knowledge you already have about what works (and doesn't work) for you.

The joy of a wonderful evening in which you don't compromise yourself but still indulge in great food and good company can be a celebration unto itself.

Vacations require the same tactics as parties. With vacations, however, you have more control because *you* pick the place, time, and companions. Read over the paragraphs above on parties. Add the strategies you'll find in the "Restaurant Tactics" chapter, and take the time to plan for your own success. It really pays and, most of all, it really works.

Surviving Spousal Sabotage

Problem

My husband says it embarrasses him when I make a fuss at a restaurant by ordering low-carb.

My wife says she'll help me diet, then cooks up a meal that's almost totally high-carb.

My husband can eat anything and stay skinny. He insists on eating cookies and junk food in front of me, knowing I can't have any, then he leaves the half-empty bags around for me to clean up!

My husband makes fun of me
being on *another* diet.
My wife buys "treats" that I can't refuse.

TroubleShooter

Spousal sabotage is as old as the history of mankind (and womankind). Sometimes it's deliberate, often it's not, but in the end, your spouse's reason for not supporting you in the way you'd like to be supported isn't as important as what you do about it.

There is a saying that has helped Richard in his past relationship get through the darkest days of sabotage and ridicule. It's made up of ten words, two letters each:

IF IT IS TO BE, IT IS UP TO ME!

We have come to understand that while a spouse can make it seem impossible to stay on your program, unless he or she actually forces high-carb food into your mouth or stands in the way of your ability to buy the low-carb food you need, you are still the one who's in control.

A negative look or word from a spouse, their failure to give you the low-carb meal they promised, their mean or insistent teasing, even their blatant disregard of the triggering effect of the sight, smell, or sound of high-carb foods are all regrettable and can be said to be unsupportive if not downright cruel. Maybe you've even used your anger about their behavior as an excuse to go off your diet. But the truth is, it was you, not your spouse, who put that piece of candy or cookie or donut in your mouth.

We know. We've been there. We share parts of our stories in the chapters "Straight Talk" and "Healthy Selfishness" so you can understand that we, too, have had to fight hard for what we wanted. But we won. And continue to win every day.

If you are a victim of spousal sabotage, intentional or otherwise, you are facing a difficult challenge that, sooner or later, we hope you will come to grips with. You may choose to confront the problem directly or you may prefer to work around it; each situation is unique and no single answer is right for everyone. The wide variety of tactics and strategies that people use to successfully handle spousal sabotage are as diverse as the people themselves, and while we would like to offer you a list of dos and don'ts, we know that, in the end, you will have to discover what works for you in your particular situation. It may be that a simple, direct conversation does the trick, or some repeated proof to your spouse that no matter how she or he tries, you won't be dissuaded from your goal. On the other hand, in some cases professional help may be the only way to get the support you need. And if your spouse refuses to change, or can't change, you may do best to just stay focused on yourself, on your own needs, on your own dreams, and most of all, on your own strength.*

In the end, remind yourself of this one important truth: IF IT IS TO BE, IT IS UP TO ME!

Breaking Free Of Weight-Loss Plateaus

Problem

What do I do if my weight loss slows to a crawl or I'm stuck at a plateau?

When I hit a plateau, I just give up.

> I must be at a plateau. I'm barely losing any weight after all this work!

TroubleShooter

Plateaus (or weight-loss slowdowns and stops) are *not* a necessary part of a low-carb weight-loss experience. In fact, one of the attractions of low-carb dieting is that the weight generally comes off at a steady pace.

If you're hitting a plateau or weight-loss slowdown, you're probably making one of three mistakes.

First, you may be expecting more of a weight loss than is humanly possible. If you anticipate losing more than one or two pounds a week on an ongoing basis, you're bound to be disappointed. You probably already know that the faster you lose weight, the more your body will slow down to prevent you

---

*For our experience see Chapter 2, "Healthy Selfishness," as well as Chapter 17, "All You Really Own."

from losing more. It's nature's way of protecting you from starving to death. Your body still thinks you're living in prehistoric times. If you're losing weight, it must mean there's a famine. Uh oh, better conserve energy. Eat the same thing that you ate last week, and you'll find yourself losing less and less, until your weight loss stops.

The best way to ensure that you stop losing weight is to lose it too fast (which can be downright unhealthy as well). Now, you probably already knew that, and you still want to lose weight quickly.

If so, keep this thought in mind. In the end, almost all low-carb dieters lose weight at exactly the same rate, whether they try to take it off quickly or at a healthy, steady pace. Though the radical low-carb dieters may lose it fast in the beginning, their weight-loss soon grinds to a halt, and though after some time they don't lose any more weight, they *do* lose their motivation to stay on their diet.

So the first thing to do if you want to avoid plateaus is to eat healthy, well-rounded meals within your program and avoid holding back food or skipping meals in an effort to speed up your weight loss, an effort that will only rebound and slow you down in the end.

The second reason for slowed or halted weight loss is the consumption of hidden carbohydrates or Carbohydrate Act-Alikes. Sugar substitutes, glutamates (under a whole variety of names), and saturated fats can slow down weight loss by keeping your body in a Saving Mode instead of a Spending Mode. For some important information on the ways in which Carbohydrate Act-Alikes can slow your weight loss, see Chapter 12, "Five Vital Clues Low-Carb Diet Doctors Miss."

Take a good look at the foods you have been eating at your low-carb meals; make certain they are on your program's low-carb list. We can all get a bit lackadaisical, letting a high-carb food, or a borderline food, slip into the great low-carb list in our minds when, in fact, it has no business being part of a low-carb meal.

Remember that even small amounts of high-carb foods at low-carb meals or the consumption of Carbohydrate Act-Alikes can slow or stop weight loss, even if you don't notice a craving rebound.

Last, but just as important, people who think that they are not losing weight quickly enough may be weighing themselves incorrectly, leading them to make inaccurate and misleading conclusions about their progress.

Getting on the scale several times a day or, even worse, only once a week, is *not* an accurate way of weighing yourself. The right way may surprise you . . . and you may find you've been losing more weight than you thought you were.

To Weigh Or Not To Weigh, That Is The Question

"Why aren't I losing weight?" "What do I have to do to break this plateau?" "Why can't I lose weight faster?"

We have found that problems with slow or stopped weight loss outnumber all others by ten to one. It's a real problem until many of these men and women learn they are already losing weight at a slow, healthy, steady pace without ever knowing it!

So before you make any changes based on the assumption that your low-carb program is not working, you need a dependable way to evaluate your progress. Some low-carb programs recommend you use ketone sticks to test whether or not you are in ketosis, that is, one of the physical states that is usually accompanied by weight loss.

> If you're on a low-carb program in which you measure ketones, you could see moderate levels of ketones on testing while the scale says you didn't lose weight.

The medical wisdom behind measuring ketones is questionable. In addition, being in ketosis does not necessarily translate into pounds lost in any consistent way. A low-carb dieter might see moderate levels of ketones on testing only to find that when they get on the scale, they haven't lost weight. On the other hand, some happy low-carb dieters have discovered that even without ketosis, they have seen the pounds drop.

Avoiding the ups and downs of ketone stick results, some dieters attempt to keep track of their weight loss by measuring the circumference of a variety of sites on their body. The greater the number of sites they measure, the greater number of inches "lost"—or so they think. Unfortunately, this is one of the most inaccurate methods of weight-loss evaluation. Unless a dieter intends to draw a permanent line around each part to be measured and compared with previous measurements, the circumference of a thigh or upper arm or hips can change greatly by simply moving the measuring tape up or down an inch.

Using clothes as an estimate of weight lost is rarely accurate enough to keep one motivated or able to judge the effectiveness of a diet, as anyone who has ever tried to use an old pair of stretched out pants or super-tight jeans as a measuring stick can attest to. And belts can be raised or lowered to bring about the desired results.

> Weighing yourself can make you anxious
> or even downright miserable.

It would seem, then, that weighing yourself offers the best choice for evaluating how well a diet is helping you bring down your weight. But here's the catch: weighing is one of the most misunderstood and quickly sacrificed elements of any weight-loss program. Because of personal histories fraught with self-blame, shame, and frustration, weighing is often accompanied by great anxiety and, for some, downright misery. But by not weighing, or by doing it in an inconsistent or illogical way, you may be disregarding an important tool for gauging the effectiveness of your diet.

So what do you do? The answer is simple. Fix the errors in

the *way* you weigh yourself that almost certainly interfere with getting an accurate evaluation of your weight-loss success.

Five Wrong Ways to Weigh Yourself

Everyone tells you the right way to weigh yourself and most people disregard it. And no wonder. The traditional "right way" of weighing yourself is wrong. It can leave you frustrated and/or elated when you may have no reason to feel either. So we figured that we would start off with the *wrong* way to weigh yourself, and explain why it can cause so many problems. We'll get to the truly right way at the end.

Here goes: If you want to be certain that you will get frustrated quickly, miss the fact that you're losing weight in a slow, steady, and healthy way, and give yourself an excuse to give up on a weight-loss program that may be working very well for you:

➤ Weigh yourself in the morning and use the number to determine how you feel about yourself for the rest of the day.
➤ Become a "scale addict" who bounces on and off the scale many times throughout the day and evening, looking for any signs of instant gratification (or punishment).
➤ Get on the scale only after a significant event, such as going to the bathroom or cheating on your eating program, and once again, let the number determine how good a person you are.
➤ Weigh yourself once a week and assume that you should see a significant weight loss with each weekly weigh-in.
➤ Develop "scale phobia" and avoid weighing yourself altogether until, finally, overcoming your fears, you face the scale, only to find that whatever weight you've lost can never equal the imagined number of pounds you think you should have lost.

Each of these self-defeating approaches to weighing yourself will almost guarantee eventual failure on any weight-loss program and, in the end, leave you feeling so bad about yourself that you are almost certain to give up trying to lose weight for a good long time. Saddest of all, your pain may be unnecessary.

The Scale Ballet: Rachael's Swan Weight

I, too, was a member of the Scale Ballet troupe. Each morning, I would rise (if not shine), go to the bathroom, then march myself to the cold metal of my judge. Placing my feet in the exact position that I had learned would produce the lightest weight, I would lean this way or that, extending my body far beyond the range of normal standing (and normal endurance), and, at times, resort to tapping the scale with my foot—moving it this way or that—all in an attempt to extract a number I could live with for the rest of the day.

> I was an expert of the Scale Ballet,
> leaning this way and that in hopes of some
> good news to get me through the day.

This was my daily moment of reckoning. I shared the results with no one, but I mulled them over throughout the day in a circle of self-blame or, on rare occasions, celebration. No matter how hard I tried, the self-blames outnumbered the celebrations by a lot, and in the end, I put the tyrant away where I would no longer have to face its nasty presence.

Only after some time had passed, and I could no longer deny that my weight was clearly out of control, did I bring the scale out once again and, stepping on it, face the horror of my transgressions. The weight went up in tens of pounds and came down, bit by bit, in single numbers if at all.

If I had known then what I know now, perhaps I might have seen that some of the diet plans I had been following had actually been working. Perhaps I might have saved myself a lot of heartache and self-blame. Perhaps not. But from those terrible experiences came a determination to help others who, in the

privacy of their own bathrooms, have felt disappointment unnecessarily and, perhaps, given up too soon.

Here, then, is what Richard and I have learned about how to
best evaluate whether or not a diet is working for you.

First Things First

Scales can be . . . Bet you finished that sentence in some interesting ways. Actually, we were going to say . . . scales can be
inaccurate. By law they are *allowed* to be inaccurate up to a certain percentage. Let's pretend, for a moment, that they are allowed to be inaccurate by only 2 percent. Not a whole lot, you
might say, but consider this: if you weigh 150 pounds and your
scale is inaccurate by 2 percent, it can be off by three pounds in
either direction.

In other words, the scale can say that you weigh 147 pounds
or 153 and still be considered accurate. That's a six-pound difference. If you weigh 200 pounds, the difference jumps to eight
pounds. So even if your weight hasn't changed at all, after a
week it could appear that you have lost or gained as much as
six or eight pounds because of the inaccuracy of the scale.

> No bathroom scale is accurate!

Deep inside, you might have already known this. How many
times have you been perfect on your diet, eaten exactly what you
were supposed to, and the scale said that you had gained weight?
And how many times have you eaten what you knew you
shouldn't have and felt the change in your weight, only to get on a
scale that said nothing had changed—or that you had *lost* weight?
You knew it then, but chances are, like all of us, you didn't trust
yourself. Maybe because you were told that "scales don't lie."
Well, they do . . . or at least, they don't always tell the truth.

In addition, the human body does not behave like a bag
of flour. It is an ever-changing, ever-in-flux biological system

altered by hormones, salt level, additives, medications, and the amount of liquid we've consumed and retained. There is only one sensible way to approach that ever-so-important measure of success we call weight loss without resorting to Scale Ballet every morning, and the depression or euphoria that follows.

> Weighing done right can be amazingly rewarding; weighing done wrong can be devastating.

When you're dealing with something as complex as the human body, numbers alone have no meaning. Scientists have learned that there is no value to individual numbers in a continually varying system; there's no way to know what is a normal variation.

However, groups of numbers averaged together can be more accurately compared. Now, don't worry. We're not about to get into higher mathematics. All we're aiming for is an *accurate* picture of how well you are doing on an ongoing basis. Weighing, done right, can be one of the most rewarding parts of a low-carb diet; weighing done wrong can be devastating.

We have developed a sane and effective way to accurately determine the rate of progress of any diet program in the world. Using a series of daily weight measurements taken under the same conditions and averaging them together (a simple, easy-to-follow explanation follows), you will avoid the gratifying ups and discouraging downs that often come with water retention, scale inaccuracies, medications, and any other variables in the human body. You will see accurate average weekly weight changes and be able to make choices in your eating program to keep you moving toward your goal.

Averaging Your Weight: Three Simple Steps

Step #1 Weigh yourself every day at about the same time with the same scale and under the same conditions. Try not to vary the time of day by more than a couple of hours. We find that the best time to weigh yourself is when you get up, after going to the bathroom, before eating or drinking anything, and before putting on any clothes. If you have some other schedule that you would like to try, feel free to do so, just keep it consistent.

Step # 2 Write down your weight on a progress chart similar to the one below. Don't promise yourself that you'll remember the figures. You know you won't. You can remember for a day, perhaps even two, but not for the whole week. Write it down.

Week Begins (Date)	Mon	Tues	Wed	Thurs	Fri	Sat	Sun	Average for the week
8/5/09	173	172	174	173	173	172	173	

Step #3 Add up the seven daily weights and divide that total by 7.* Then compare the average with the average from the week before.

That's it—all it takes to get an accurate picture of how you are doing on your program and whether your low-carb diet is working for you. We generally recommend that you keep track for about three weeks before drawing any conclusions.

It's All in the Details

The saying goes that it's all in the details. When it comes to measuring weight, we couldn't agree more. Consider the weight chart above. Adding up the seven days you get a total of 1,210 pounds.

Dividing 1,210 by the number of weigh-ins for the week, in this case 7 (you can use a calculator if you wish), and you get

---

*That is, divide by 7 assuming you have seven measurements. If you missed a day, divide by the total number of days for which you do have a weight. For example, if you only have five weights for the week, divide the total by 5, if you have six weights for the week, divide the total by 6.

172.85 pounds, rounded off to 172.9, which is your average weight for the week.

Look at the first week compared to a second week.

Week Begins Date	Mon	Tues	Wed	Thurs	Fri	Sat	Sun	Average for the week
8/5/09	173	172	174	173	173	172	173	172.9
8/12/09	170	173	170	172	174	171	171	171.6

Even though the numbers don't look very different when viewed day to day, you can see that *on average*, this person has lost 1.3 pounds from week one to week two—a weight loss that most health care professionals would agree is ideal. Success— despite daily weights that gave the impression there was no weight lost at all!

> Individual daily or weekly weights make it look like you're losing weight when you're not, or they can do the opposite.

Daily or weekly weigh-ins can drive you crazy or, even worse, rob you of the very success and happiness you have been seeking for so long.

It's essential that you keep in mind that your daily weight can move up or down in reaction to:

➤ Eating out
➤ Sudden changes in health, such as a cold or flu, or the use of certain medications
➤ Hormonal changes
➤ Stress

One of the most important things that you can do for yourself is to leave behind the old rules and expectations that have failed you in the past. Be realistic and content with a moderate rate of weight loss. Instant gratification is not your friend. Don't listen to its insistent demand. Remember that if you consistently lose one pound a week, at the end of a year you will have lost fifty-two pounds!

So this time do it differently:

➤ Set a realistic goal for how fast you will lose weight and what your final result will be. Consult with your doctor and determine a target weight at which you will be healthy and happy.

➤ Don't allow yourself to be influenced by the temporary effects of salt or other additives in your foods (especially glutamates) that can cause a temporary jump in your weight.* You need to be strong enough to fight off the old voices of self-blame and work for the long term.

➤ Stay focused on your program, keep averaging your weights, and don't let anyone dissuade you from your goal. Put yourself first and give yourself all the support you'd give any good friend who was trying hard to succeed. If you don't, who will?

➤ Take the words "cheat" and "treat" out of your vocabulary. You are either following your program or you aren't. If you go off your program, figure out what went wrong and do it right next time. If it takes more than one try, fine. Each time you try, you'll learn something new.

➤ Most of all, let go of the self-blame of the past and stay focused on the wonderful future that lies ahead.

If I Just Lose This Many Pounds for This Many Weeks: Rachael's Hard-Won Lesson†

This section would not be complete without addressing one of the most important aspects of measuring weight and the one

---

*For more information on glutamates, see our chapter "Five Vital Clues Low-Carb Diet Doctors Miss."

†We both share our personal stories in our book *The Carbohydrate Addict's LifeSpan Program.*

that almost no one ever listens to (though they end up paying the price for it in the end).

The human body is a very clever arrangement of systems that react to the environment. Do something too quickly and the body will adjust to protect itself. For instance, if you lose weight too quickly, the body will do everything in its power to slow or stop the weight loss.

The old caution that you should not lose weight too quickly is not just something people say to make you feel better—it's true! As a scientist, I was well aware of the research that had repeatedly shown that the best rate of weight loss is no more than a pound and a half to two pounds a week. But I had ignored it all my life (while wondering why each drop in weight was often followed by my weight loss coming to a screeching stop).

When I gained weight beyond what my bathroom scale could measure, I knew I had to give up on my "I've got to take it off as fast as I can so I can live with myself" approach to weight loss. At the same time, I faced the very sobering thought that since I weighed three hundred pounds, it would take me almost two years to get down to my goal weight if I lost at the recommended rate. I also knew, not only from my reading but from a lifetime of experience, that when I lost weight any faster than that, my body would balk and the weight loss would slow down or stop no matter how hard I tried.

So, for once in my life, I stopped counting the weeks it would take me to get thin and concentrated, instead, on staying on my program. I didn't starve myself in order to wring out one more extra pound of lost weight at the end of the week. I just ate in the ways I had come to realize would cut my cravings and take off the weight and the pounds came off at a slow and steady pace—on the *average* of one or two pounds per week.

In the end, it took me two years to lose one hundred and sixty-five pounds. To others, that may seem like a long time, but I enjoyed every step along the way. (I actually needed the time to adjust to the "new me" that was emerging, as well.) Now I've had over twenty years (so far!) to enjoy my weight loss, so I guess it was time well spent after all.

Richard lost his forty-five pounds in almost exactly the same way. It took him about six months, but he, too, has kept if off without struggle for over two decades.

Take the time to get it right. Losing weight isn't a race. Rather it's a long-term process of gradually integrating new ways of eating into your daily life, so that they become pleasurable and permanent parts of a healthier way of living.

Losing weight requires overcoming obstacles—both inside and outside yourself—ferreting out the solutions to puzzling mysteries, and developing patterns of behavior that put your needs first. Making changes—even simple, easy ones—takes time, and so does losing weight. Yet by mastering small changes, and building one change upon another, you'll be surprised to find how much your patterns of eating change—and how much closer you are to achieving success!

Chapter 16

RESTAURANT TACTICS

Getting What You Want, When You
Want It, Without Feeling Guilty

We're going to look at "the challenge of the restaurant" in a whole new way. Instead of giving you a list of dos and don'ts on restaurant eating, let's see what you already know and go from there.

> How many Diet Defeaters can you spot?

Here's your restaurant challenge. Your goal is to stay on your low-carb diet while being served a deliciously prepared meal with a minimal amount of stress. How many Diet Defeaters can you spot with the following story:

It's eight o'clock on a Saturday night and you're having dinner with two friends, Jennifer and Kevin. The restaurant is Jennifer's newest discovery and she's been dying to get you to join her here for weeks. Jennifer is usually on time and Kevin is almost always late, as you and Jennifer both know.

You show up at the agreed-on hour and are glad for a little time alone with Jennifer before Kevin's arrival, to talk to Jennifer about a possible investment opportunity that could help your sister's husband.

> Your day has been crazy; you never
> thought you'd get it all done.

Your day has been frantic, with a million tasks that you had to finish before you left for the restaurant, but you manage to arrive on time.

Checking in with the maître d', you find that Jennifer has neither arrived nor called. She might have left a message on your cell phone, which you brought but forgot to recharge.

As you are deciding how to contact her, Jennifer arrives in a flurry, talking nonstop about her breakup with her latest boyfriend.

> Kevin is always late. They won't
> seat you until he arrives.

While she goes on about the details, the maître d' informs you that it is the policy of the restaurant to wait until all parties have arrived before seating you at your table. He expresses his apology, however, and offers you and Jennifer a drink on the house.

You decide it would be impolite to decline (after all, the drink is free), so you accept, having a tall, cool strawberry margarita that you hadn't planned on.

> You've earned the right to a
> nice drink; besides, it's free!

You tell yourself that you deserve the drink, especially in light of the fact that you are going to have to put up with yet another of Jennifer's "boyfriend stories." You sip the margarita slowly, trying to figure how you might turn the conversation to your sister's husband and the investment opportunity you promised your sister you'd bring up. As the minutes pass, you begin to munch on the bar snacks well within your reach.

By the time Kevin arrives and you are seated at your table, it's almost nine o'clock. You are starved. Waiting for the waiter, you nibble on the ultra-thin cracker bread, telling yourself that if it's that thin, it can't have many carbs. Besides, you promise yourself you will have a perfectly "legal" low-carb meal to make up for it.

When you open the menu, however, you're floored. The prices are twice what you expected to pay. Though you are upset about the price, you force down your concern and order what you assume will be a good low-carb way to go, no matter what the cost.

As each course arrives, however, you're in for another surprise: gourmet dining at its worst, with portions that are apparently fit only for the nutritional needs of a four-year-old. Your salad is nothing but a few leaves of multicolored greens, bitter to the taste and topped with a sickeningly sweet dressing that is clearly not low-carb. A miniscule filet follows, perched in the center of a large plate, beautifully decorated with drizzles of color and a few tiny baby vegetables. This meal does not a satisfying low-carb dinner make! For a moment, you consider ordering a second meal, but knowing that Kevin would die of embarrassment, and considering the cost, you force down the disappointing meal.

> A tiny meal at twice the price. You
> force down the food and the feelings.

You decline dessert, resolute to stay on your diet (and avoid an unnecessary expense), but when you get home, you hit the refrigerator at full throttle, downing more carbs than you can count. You fall asleep feeling like a failure, promising yourself that you'll never do that again and vaguely remembering that you've been through this before.

* * *

Okay, how many Diet Defeaters did you spot and what could have been done about them? Let's compare notes:

It's eight o'clock on a Saturday night and you're having dinner with two friends, Jennifer and Kevin.

Eight o'clock on Saturday night is probably the worst time to try and get what you want at a busy restaurant. The restaurant is running full steam—no time for special requests—and by that late hour, you're too hungry to care about anything but getting some food in your mouth.

The restaurant is Jennifer's newest discovery and she's been dying to get you to join her here for weeks.

Letting someone else choose the restaurant is almost certain to ensure that you will go off your low-carb diet, be stressed or disappointed, or all of the above. When it comes to deciding where to eat, *you* make the choice. Put yourself and your goals first. To others, the choice of restaurant is just a bit of fun; to you, it's a matter of health, appearance, and self-esteem.

If you like, give friends a choice of several restaurants you know you can count on for a good and satisfying low-carb meal. Let them choose, if you like—but only from your basic list.

Kevin is almost always late, as you and Jennifer both know.

If you must eat with people who are not punctual, make contingency plans. "Look, I'm going to be starving by then so if you aren't there by such-and-such a time, I'm going to order and get started on my meal. That way you won't feel pressured and I won't be dying to eat!"

Better yet, don't make restaurant plans with people who can't be counted on to show up on time. Take care of yourself first. When you think about it, isn't that what they're doing?

You show up at the agreed-on hour and are glad for a little time alone with Jennifer before Kevin's arrival, to talk to Jennifer about a possible investment opportunity that could help your sister's husband.

If your goal is to stick to your low-carb diet, then sticking to it has to be your top priority. Putting other demands on yourself while trying to navigate the treacherous waters of restaurant dining can be a setup for failure.

When faced with trying to accomplish two or more tasks at the same time, your body is far more likely to release stress hormones and, in turn, insulin surges, making it almost impossible to stay focused on eating low-carb.

Over the years, we have found that some people are able to be productive at a business meal without straying from their low-carb commitments, but to a person if they have to choose between paying attention to their low-carb eating and trying to accomplish some other goal during the meal, sticking to their diet always wins out, hands down.

To succeed at your low-carb diet when dining at restaurants (or anywhere else), you're going to have to become a little selfish. (See our "Healthy Selfishness" chapter if you need a bit of encouragement.) We tell ourselves we have one job: staying on our diet. All else comes and goes and, in many cases, so do the people.

Your day has been frantic with a million tasks that you had to finish before you left for the restaurant, but you manage to arrive on time. Checking in with the maître d', you find that Jennifer has neither arrived nor called. She might have left a message on your cell phone, which you brought but forgot to recharge.

You are showing every sign of a perfectly normal life that's out of control and bound for diet failure. You are trying to juggle so many tasks that you are bound to drop at least one. Unfortunately, the first to go is usually your low-carb diet. After all, there's usually a part of us that's looking for an excuse to take a vacation from it anyway. In addition, the other demands we are juggling generally have to be taken care of *now*, and other people are usually counting on us to get them right.

So is it any wonder that the first casualty of an impossible schedule is the one thing that would make us feel the best and give us the most joy in return?

Most of us try to continue to do it all, however. Until you reach the point where you can put your hand in the air and yell "Stop! This whole thing is just too much. I'm number one and my eating and my weight take top priority."—until you say that and *mean* it and *keep* meaning it—whatever comes along will push aside all your good intentions and convince you that you will never succeed.

We urge you to do it, to stop being the "good" person that everyone can count on. Losing weight is about much more than changing your eating or your lifestyle. It's about putting yourself first and giving your needs and dreams the seriousness and respect they deserve.

As you are deciding how to contact her, Jennifer arrives in a flurry, talking nonstop about her breakup with her latest boyfriend. While she goes on about the details, the maître d' informs you that it is the policy of the restaurant to wait until all parties have arrived before seating you at your table. He expresses his apology, however, and offers you and Jennifer a drink on the house.

Here is where almost every restaurant diet failure can be avoided. Had you chosen the restaurant, you would have been familiar with its policies and staff. With a little forethought, you would not have combined a chronically late dinner companion with a policy that would leave you stranded in the bar until he happened to wander in. Or, knowing the staff, you might have asked to have the policy waived.

Even without knowing the policy or staff, a simple call ahead to the restaurant could have given you the opportunity to speak with someone who could make an exception in your case or would have alerted you to the fact that you needed to choose a different restaurant.

Of greatest importance, however, is the attitude of caring and concern you must develop for yourself, your willingness to do what it takes to get you the setting, food, and experience of eating that you need in order to stay on your program.

If you had a child who was allergic to some food product, you would not simply show up at a restaurant and expect to get that child what he or she needed, and if it were not available, simply make do. The same would be true for your mate, or a friend, or even a guest. You might even extend this care to a pet with special needs, calling ahead to make certain a kennel had the food that was needed to keep him/her healthy. Isn't it strange that we resist doing as much for ourselves?

You decide it would be impolite to decline (after all, the drink is free), so you accept, having a tall, cool strawberry margarita that you hadn't planned on.

Free food or drink has an almost irresistible appeal. Just because it's free, people eat food they would never *think* of paying for, even when it doesn't taste good or when it is decidedly not on their eating program. We don't understand it completely. Richard isn't affected by the offer of free food, but I'm attracted as if to a thousand-pound magnet. Whatever the reason, watch out for the allure of free food or drink.

If you find yourself sorely tempted by free food, we recommend the following: first, put some distance between yourself and the offer. Get out. Go to the bathroom. Make a phone call. Anything to get some time to think.

Then, talk out loud to yourself. Whether in a bathroom stall or on the phone or by writing it out, talk to yourself. Ask yourself how much the food is really worth and if you could afford to buy yourself something else that might be much better for you in every way.

Finally, make a plan that involves an alternative pleasure. Go back and have a cup of iced tea, knowing that later that evening you'll treat yourself to a more satisfying choice.

Don't expect to just give up the freebies in hopes of feeling self-righteous. That doesn't work for long. Give yourself something good in exchange. That way you reap two rewards: the gift you've traded the free food for and the pleasure of staying on your program.

You tell yourself that you deserve the drink, especially in light of the fact that you are going to have to put up with yet another of Jennifer's "boyfriend stories." You sip the margarita slowly, trying to figure how you might turn the conversation to your sister's husband and the investment opportunity you promised your sister you'd bring up. As the minutes pass, you begin to munch on the bar snacks well within your reach.

We all use food as a reward. Scientists use it to train and test lab animals. Parents use it to bribe their kids into behaving well. All kinds of people reward themselves with food in exchange for doing a range of tasks that they don't particularly want to do.

For most people, using food as a reward is a harmless "trick," one among a whole bag of treats they offer themselves for a job well done. But for some people with a weight or eating problem, especially those with high levels of insulin, food can become the primary source of pleasure.

If food has become your primary source of pleasure, and you use it to bribe yourself into doing onerous tasks that are so "distasteful" to you that you can only "swallow" them with food, you may be using food to cover up some other problem in your professional or personal life that needs to be addressed. Do you want to put up with situations that go beyond what should be acceptable to you, simply because you're rewarding yourself with the food you want more than anything else?

If you can stop the internal bribery, if you can stop using food as your sole reward, your whole life could change, and a whole new you could emerge.

By the time Kevin arrives and you are seated at your table, it's almost nine o'clock. You are starved. Waiting for the waiter, you nibble on the ultra-thin cracker bread, telling yourself that if it's that thin, it can't have many carbs. Besides, you promise yourself you will have a perfectly "legal" low-carb meal to make up for it.

We are funny, aren't we? If we're "good" on our diets all day, we go off the diet to reward ourselves. If we cheat on our diet, we convince ourselves it will be okay as long as we don't do all the damage we *could* do.

Stop rationalizing, making deals, or making promises about your diet, your eating, or your weight (to yourself or others). They are keeping you from seeing that you have put yourself in an impossible situation and that you've got to make some changes. You'd do far better to realize what barriers you've allowed to be thrown in your path, figure out how to avoid them in the future, give yourself the *right* to do it differently next time, and, oh yes, have a perfectly "legal" low-carb meal as well.

When you open the menu, however, you're floored. The prices are twice what you expected to pay. Though you

*are upset about the price, you force down your concern
and order what you assume will be a good low-carb way
to go, no matter what the cost.*

More stress, more insulin, and your ability to control your
eating has become almost nil. Your choice of restaurant or a call
ahead would have solved it all.

*As each course arrives, however, you're in for another
surprise: gourmet dining at its worst, with portions that
are apparently fit only for the nutritional needs of a four-
year-old. Your salad is nothing but a few leaves of multicolored greens, bitter to the taste and topped with a
sickeningly sweet dressing that is clearly not low-carb. A
miniscule filet follows, perched in the center of a large
plate, beautifully decorated with drizzles of color and a
few tiny baby vegetables. This meal does not a satisfying
low-carb dinner make! For a moment, you consider ordering a second meal, but knowing that Kevin would die of
embarrassment, and considering the cost, you force down
the disappointing meal.*

Don't do it! We can't tell you how much we hate to see this
happen. This is your body and your life. You cannot throw it all
away just because you might "embarrass" someone. A true
friend will want what's best for you; if your dinner companion
isn't a true friend, why are you trying to please him?

And if the meal isn't right for you, if it doesn't meet the requirements of your eating program or it simply doesn't taste
good, don't force it down! Haven't we all forced down enough
in our lives?

*You decline dessert, resolute to stay on your diet (and
avoid an unnecessary expense), but when you get home,
you hit the refrigerator at full throttle, downing more
carbs than you can count. You fall asleep feeling like a
failure, promising yourself that you'll never do that again
and vaguely remembering that you've been through this
before.*

Of course you blew it! Look at the setup that taking care of
other people set in motion. Your feelings of failure, however,
can keep you from seeing that the way out lies in your hands.

Take yourself and your dreams seriously. Set the rules—and stick to them. Don't put the preferences of others before your own needs and goals.

Choose the time, place, and people, make arrangements beforehand, and never force down the food or the feelings.

Each time you take care of yourself, give yourself what you need, and refuse to succumb to guilt for making sane, healthy choices, you will be changing, evolving into a person who reaches out for the life you want, and gets it. For those of us who have struggled to find a balance between taking care of others and taking care of ourselves, success is about a whole lot more than just food; it can change your whole life for the better. And, after all, isn't that what you wanted?

Chapter 17

ALL YOU REALLY OWN

For both of us, the most nerve-racking part of any action movie is when the hero and heroine finally understand what is happening, but despite their desperate struggle against their enemies, they appear to be headed for disaster. We hold our breath and hope that they're granted one more chance to make it right.

Unlike the movies, real life almost always gives us another chance. Conventional wisdom says that each of us learns too little too late, but we disagree. We think that learning is the path, and the only challenge is to put what we've learned into action.

The real question, then, is not how you slip up, miscalculate, or even downright mess up your life, or your diet, but rather how you pick yourself up, brush yourself off, and start again—not from the beginning but from where you left off.

Let go of your fears of success or failure. Embrace the fact that—no matter what—you haven't given up. Love yourself for that!

Value your mistakes. They are the best foundation upon which to construct your success.

Listen to the inner voice that tells you not to give up. When you argue with it, disregard it, or ridicule it, it grows silent. Nurture it and let it know that it is loved, and it will grow strong, until one day it will guide you loudly and clearly.

That voice led us into a new life, and it can do the same for you.

Though others may not understand your perseverance, it's all you may ever own in this unpredictable world.

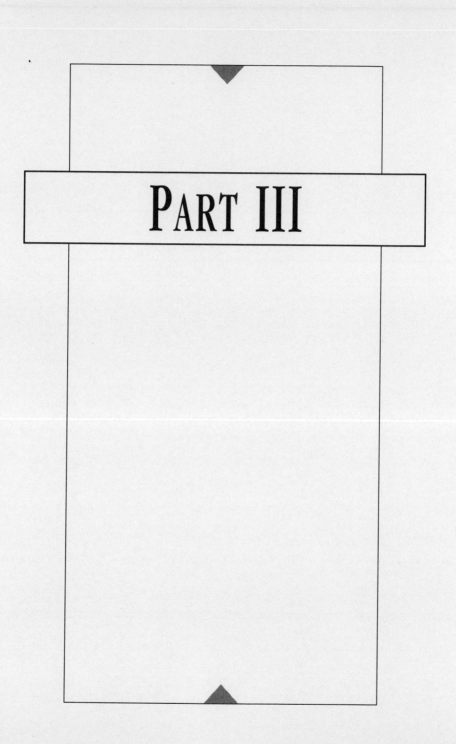

PART III

Chapter 18

RESCUE RECIPES

WARM SPINACH CHEESE DIP

Prep Time: 5 minutes   *Cook Time: 25 minutes*   *Makes 3 cups*

We can hardly believe how good this dip is. We bring it to parties and dinners and make it for ourselves as a special treat. It's a wonderful served up as a warm appetizer or an amazing snack.

  2 8-oz. pkg. cream cheese, softened, cut into 1-inch blocks
  1 10-oz. pkg. frozen spinach, thawed, drained
  ½ cup heavy cream or sour cream
  ½ cup grated Parmesan or Romano cheese
  1 clove garlic, minced

Combine the ingredients in a food processor or beat with an electric mixer.

Spoon into a 9-inch pie plate.

Bake at 350°F. for about 25 minutes.

Serve warm with low-carb vegetables and enjoy!

CREPES IN A MINUTE

Prep Time: 10 minutes   *Cook Time: 10 minutes*
Makes 4 large crepes

Ready when you need them, these quick-fixers turn any low-carb leftover into a grab-and-go treat. We love them filled with tuna salad or as taco crepes, filled with browned hamburger, shredded lettuce, and cheese.

4   eggs
4   tablespoons heavy cream
    Salt, black pepper, cayenne, oregano, or sweet dried basil as
      desired, depending on the low-carb stuffing.
2   tablespoons butter or olive oil

Combine the ingredients in a medium bowl.
Heat a small amount of butter or olive oil in an 8-inch non-stick frying pan.
Pour about ¼ of the mixture into the pan, swirling quickly to cover the bottom with a thin layer.
Cook for only a few minutes, until the bottom is brown. Flip gently and lightly brown the other side. Remove from the pan.
Repeat for each remaining crepe.

LOW-CARB LASAGNA

Prep Time: 20 minutes   *Time: 40 minutes*   *Serves 4*

We love this lasagna because it's as hearty and satisfying as the high-carb variety. It has "layers of pleasure" we enjoy when we want something really filling.

1   **pound lean ground beef**
2   **tablespoons olive oil**
¼   **small onion, diced**
½   **green pepper, diced**
1   **clove garlic, crushed**
1   **tablespoon oregano**
1   **egg, beaten**
8   **ounces ricotta cheese**
    Salt and pepper
3   **portobello mushrooms, sliced thin horizontally**
8   **ounces spinach (or other low-carb vegetable), steamed**
4   **ounces mozzarella cheese, shredded**
¼   **cup Parmesan cheese, shredded**

Brown the meat in about 2 tablespoons olive oil.

When the meat is nearly done, add the onion and the green pepper and sauté until the onion softens.

Add the garlic and continue cooking until the onions brown. Add the oregano and remove from heat.

In a medium bowl, combine the egg and the ricotta together. Add salt and pepper as desired.

Preheat the oven to 325°F.

Grease a loaf pan with olive oil. Spread ½ of the meat mixture in the bottom of the pan. Top with a layer of sliced portobello mushrooms followed by a layer of the ricotta mixture. Top with spinach (or other vegetable), then a layer using ½ of the cheeses.

Cover with the remaining meat mixture and top with the remaining cheese.

Bake at 325° for about 40 minutes.

Remove when the meat is thoroughly cooked and the cheese is bubbly and starting to brown.

SHRIMP DIJON

Prep Time: 5 minutes   Cook Time: 10 to 12 minutes   Serves 4

We make this dish as an appetizer and spice it up according to our mood by adding a bit of Hungarian paprika or cayenne to taste.

    1 **pound large shrimp, raw, cleaned with tails left on**
    ⅛ **cup dry white wine (optional)***
    4 **tablespoons olive oil**
   10 **sprigs fresh parsley, chopped**
    2 **tablespoons Dijon mustard**
       Black pepper, salt, paprika, or cayenne, as desired.

Preheat the oven to 425°F.

Place the shrimp in an oiled baking dish.

Combine the wine, oil, parsley, and mustard in a blender; purée.

Add black pepper, salt, paprika, or cayenne, as desired.

Pour the purée over the shrimp.

Place the baking dish in the preheated oven.

Bake 10 to 12 minutes, turning once and basting while cooking; season to taste.

---

*Optional ingredient. Include only if permitted on your particular low-carb or controlled-carb eating program.

CREAM CHEESE CLOUD*

Prep Time: 3 minutes   *Cook Time: 0 minutes*   *Serves 2*

A special treat that makes us feel decadent. The dash of cinnamon makes it complete.

- ½ cup sour cream
- 3 ounces cream cheese
- 2 tablespoons brandy (for optimal taste)
  Dash of cinnamon

Place the sour cream and cheese in a mixing bowl or blender. Add the brandy and mix.

Serve in a glass dessert dish, topped with a sprinkle of cinnamon.

HEARTY CHICKEN WITH MUSHROOMS

Prep Time: 6 minutes   *Cook Time: 15 to 20 minutes*   *Serves 2*

An old family recipe. We usually serve it on Sunday, as a late afternoon dinner, and sometimes with guests.

- 1 tablespoon butter
- 1 tablespoon olive oil
- 1 teaspoon green peppercorns in vinegar
- 1 chicken breast split in halves, skinned and boned
- 1 cup chopped celery
- 2 cups mushroom caps, cleaned
- 1 cup chicken stock*
  Salt and pepper, to taste

---

*Make this recipe only if 2 tablespoons of brandy is permitted on your particular low-carb or controlled-carb eating program.

Heat the butter in a skillet.

Add the green peppercorns. Stir 1 minute.

Place the half breasts in the skillet and cook over medium heat until the chicken becomes tannish in color, about 3 minutes. Turn and cook until thoroughly cooked.

Add the celery and mushrooms to the sides of pan, leaving the chicken breasts in the center.

Pour in ½ cup of the chicken stock, cover the pan with a partially open cover, and simmer for about 10 minutes over low heat.

Add the remaining ½ cup of stock to the pan. Bring to a boil and let cook to reduce and thicken the sauce.

Add salt and pepper to taste.

WINGED SALVATION

Prep Time: 12 minutes   *Cook Time: 1 hour*   *Serves 2*

We cook up a batch of these, keep them handy, then grab 'em when we're on the go.

12 **chicken wings**
 1 **cup Parmesan cheese, dry or fresh, grated**
 1 **teaspoon garlic powder**
 1 **teaspoon dried chopped parsley**
 ½ **cup olive oil**
 2 **tablespoons melted butter, cooled**
    Black pepper, to taste, if desired
    Cayenne pepper, to taste, if desired

---

*If you're using prepared stock, check the label for high-carb additives and other Carbohydrate Act-Alikes.

Preheat the oven to 350°F.

Wash the wings and pat them dry with fresh paper towels.

Place them on a lightly oiled cookie sheet or broiler pan. (Wash your hands after.)

In a large bowl or pot, combine the cheese, garlic powder, and parsley. Add black or cayenne pepper as desired. Mix very well.

Dip the wings in a mixture of the olive oil and melted butter, then into the cheese mixture.

Arrange them on a baking dish. Discard the remainder of the mixture.

Bake, uncovered, for 50 minutes. Raise the oven temperature to 375°F for another 10 minutes.

Serve warm or cold.

Variation: We use chunks of white-meat chicken to make our own chicken "nuggets."

TAIWANESE SESAME PORK WITH GARLIC CREAM SAUCE

Prep Time: 5 minutes   *Cook Time: 20 minutes*   *Serves 2*

Gourmet taste and low-carb legal. We serve it when we have guests but always make extra for the next day.

- **3   to 4 pork chops, center cut, thin**
- **3   tablespoons olive oil**
- **2   tablespoons butter**
- **2   cloves garlic, finely chopped (or ¼ to ½ teaspoon garlic powder)**
- **1   tablespoon sesame seeds (optional)***
- **3   ounces cream cheese, softened**
- **⅓   cup heavy cream**
- **1   teaspoon chives, dried and chopped**

---

*Optional ingredient. Include only if permitted on your particular low-carb or controlled-carb eating program.

Place the chops in oil in a skillet.

Cook over medium heat until well browned on one side. Turn and continue to cook until well done throughout.

While the pork is cooking, melt the butter in a small skillet over low heat. Cook the garlic in the butter until it softens, about 3 minutes. Reduce heat to low.

Sprinkle the garlic with the sesame seeds, stir, and continue to cook for 1 minute. Reduce heat to very low.

Stir the cream cheese and cream into the garlic mixture. Cook about 1 minute, stirring constantly, until smooth and hot. Stir in the chives.

Remove the pork from the pan, allowing the oil to drip off.

Cover with the cream sauce. Serve.

CHICKEN ATHENA

Prep Time: 15 minutes   *Cook Time: 40 minutes*   *Serves 4*

Our favorite Greek restaurant serves a chicken dish we have tried to duplicate at home for years. It's simple but delicious. We always make twice what we need so we're sure of having leftovers.

  2 **tablespoons olive oil**
  4 **chicken breast fillets, boneless, skinless**
  ½ **cup Parmesan cheese**
  ¼ **cup crumbled feta cheese**
  2 **tablespoons butter, melted**
  1 **package frozen spinach, thawed**

Preheat the oven to 400°F.

Lightly grease a baking dish with olive oil.

Place each chicken breast between 2 sheets of plastic wrap or in a plastic ziplock bag and flatten it with a meat mallet until ¼-inch thick.

Dredge each chicken breast in Parmesan cheese on both sides.

Evenly divide the feta cheese among all chicken breasts. Place the cheese on one end and fold the chicken in half.

Place the chicken in the oiled baking dish and top with the melted butter.

Bake uncovered for 30 minutes.

While the chicken is cooking, heat the spinach according to package directions, until warmed. Drain well.

When the chicken is thoroughly cooked, place it on top of the spinach mound. Drizzle over the chicken the melted butter remaining in the baking dish.

SICILIAN SEA SCALLOP SCAMPI

Prep Time: 10 minutes   *Cook Time: 15 minutes*   *Serves 3*

We love this dish as an appetizer or main meal. We often serve more than one protein at a meal because we enjoy a variety of tastes. This is one of our longtime favorites that couples well with a shrimp dish at the same meal.

1   **tablespoon butter**
3   **tablespoons olive oil**
4   **cloves garlic, chopped (or equivalent in garlic powder)**
1   **pound sea scallops**
½   **teaspoon oregano, dried, chopped**
1   **teaspoon dried basil**
    Salt and pepper
¼   **cup lemon juice**
¼   **cup Marsala wine (optional)***

*Optional ingredient. Include only if permitted on your particular low-carb or controlled-carb eating program.

Melt the butter in a skillet over medium heat. Add the olive oil and diced garlic (or garlic powder). Sauté until the garlic softens and the mixture is warm.

Add the scallops and sauté until fully cooked.

Add the oregano and basil. Simmer 2 to 3 minutes.

Add salt and pepper to taste.

Using a slotted spoon, remove the scallops to a serving dish.

Add the lemon juice and Marsala wine to the pan and simmer. If wine is not use, add paprika and/or cayenne pepper to taste. Pour the sauce over the scallops.

Cover and let the flavors infuse for a few minutes before serving.

NEW ORLEANS CRUSTLESS QUICHE

Prep Time: 7 minutes   *Cook Time: 45 minutes*   *Serves 6*

This is the first dish we made for Alex* (using quite a bit of cayenne at his request). Since it opened up a whole world of vegetable eating for him, we named it after his home town.

1 **cup light cream**
1 **cup cheese (cheddar, Swiss, or American, low-fat or regular)**
1 **pound sea scallops**
1 **teaspoon olive oil**
1 **package frozen spinach, thawed, drained**
   Cayenne pepper, if desired
2 **teaspoons sweet dried basil**
3 **eggs (*no* low-fat substitute)**
   Salt and black pepper

Preheat the oven to 325°F.

Oil the sides and bottom of a 9-inch pie pan.

---

*You'll find Alex's story, "Anything But Vegetables" in the chapter titled "Day #2: Back in Control" in this book.

In a medium saucepan, heat the cream until scalded. Reduce heat.

Stir in the grated cheese until completely melted.

Squeeze the liquid from the spinach and stir in.

Add cayenne to taste and the basil.

Remove from heat and allow to cool for 5 minutes.

Add one egg at a time, mixing thoroughly after each addition.

Add salt and pepper as desired.

Pour the mixture into the pie pan, place in the oven, and bake until the custard is set (45 to 50 minutes).

Serve warm from the oven or cold, as a special leftover that's always satisfying. Freeze in individual servings for easy breakfasts.

INSTANT BREAKFAST SAUSAGE

Prep Time: 5 minutes   *Cook Time: 15 minutes*   *Serves 4*

We make up a batch of these and stock them in the freezer. When we want a special treat for breakfast (or anytime), we put a patty or two on one of the Crepes in a Minute (recipe in this section), then add some cheese while the sausage is warm. Yum!

  1 **pound ground turkey**
 ½ **tablespoon dried sage**
 ½ **teaspoon ground pepper**
 ¼ **teaspoon ground cloves**
 ¼ **teaspoon nutmeg**
 ½ **teaspoon sweet dried basil**
 ¼ **teaspoon ground cloves**
 ¼ **teaspoon nutmeg**
  4 **tablespoons olive oil**

In a large bowl, combine and mix the turkey, well ground, and all the herbs.

Divide the mixture into 8 equal portions. Shape it into thin patties.

Place the oil in a large frying pan over moderate heat.

When the pan is hot, brown the patties on both sides (making sure that they are cooked thoroughly).

Serve warm or freeze for a quick-fix breakfast. Top with melted cheese or wrap in lettuce leaves spiced with mustard.

YOU-ADD-THE-EXTRAS BASIC CREAMY DIP AND DRESSING

Prep Time: 5 minutes Cook Time: 0 minutes Makes about 1 cup

Limited only by your imagination. We add whatever low-carb leftovers spark our fancy, including (but not limited to) tuna, chicken, horseradish, or Parmesan cheese.

3 oz. package cream cheese
¼ cup olive oil
½ teaspoon garlic powder
½ teaspoon ared mustard
   Salt and ground black pepper

Cut the cream cheese into small chunks. Gradually add the oil, beating until smooth.

Add the garlic, mustard, and salt and pepper (to taste). Beat until blended completely.

Add your favorite spices, hot sauce, cayenne, Parmesan cheese, horseradish, and/or a bit of sautéed and browned beef. Be as creative as you like.

Chill and enjoy as dip with low-carb vegetables. It's especially good with raw green beans or celery sticks or as a luscious (and dependable) salad dressing.

MUSHROOM GARLIC DIP

Prep Time: 6 minutes   *Cook Time: 4 minutes*
Makes about 1½ cups

We love this recipe because it works as a dip, dressing, or marinade and makes almost any low-carb protein or vegetable taste special.

 1 **cup mushrooms, cleaned, dried, sliced**
 ⅔ **cup olive oil**
 ½ **teaspoon mustard powder**
 ½ **teaspoon garlic powder**
 ⅓ **cup white vinegar**
    Salt and pepper, to taste

In a small skillet, sauté the mushrooms in two tablespoons of the olive oil until browned.

In a blender or mixer bowl, add the mushrooms and olive oil from the skillet. Add the mustard and garlic powder.

Add the remaining oil and the vinegar and salt and pepper, to taste.

Blend or stir until thoroughly mixed. Refrigerate.

Use as salad dressing, low-carb vegetable dip, or marinade for chicken or fish.

OLD-FASHIONED BUTTERMILK DRESSING

Prep Time: 2 minutes   *Cook Time: 0 minutes*   *Makes 1½ cups*

We bring this dressing, along with a big salad, to barbecues. We add some low-carb protein from the grill and we're all set.

1   cup buttermilk (regular or low-fat)
¼   cup sour cream (regular or low-fat)
¼   cup fresh parsley or dried equivalent
¼   teaspoon salt (or salt substitute)
½   teaspoon dry mustard
¼   teaspoon black pepper
    Sesame seeds and poppy seeds, to taste, as allowed on your
    program.*

Place all the ingredients into a large bowl.
Combine with a whisk until smooth.
Cover and refrigerate.

POLYNESIAN LEMON-LIME STEAK

Prep Time: 4 minutes   *Cook Time: 26 minutes*   *Serves 4*

We were first served this delicately balanced dish in Australia,
at the home of a Japanese dignitary who had requested that his
Hawaiian cook prepare her signature dish for us. We loved it
and begged her for the recipe, which she was happy to share. It
was not until we returned home and opened the envelope that
we realized it was written in *Hawaiian*.

4   large rib-eye steaks
⅛   cup lemon juice (or zest)
⅛   cup lime juice (or zest)
3   teaspoons olive oil
2   cloves garlic, minced
½   teaspoon dried sweet basil
½   teaspoon cayenne pepper
½   teaspoon Teriyaki sauce (optional)*

---

*Optional ingredient. Include only if permitted on your particular low-carb or
controlled-carb eating program.

Arrange the steaks in a single layer in a broiler pan.

Combine the remaining ingredients in a medium bowl and mix well.

Pour half of the mixture over the steak. Hold the remainder.

In nice weather, cook the steak on an outdoor grill, until cooked through, turning and brushing each side with the lemon-lime mixture. In bad weather, broil in the oven until thoroughly cooked, brushing the other side with the remaining lemon-lime mixture.

TUNA-STUFFED MUSHROOMS

Prep Time: 5 minutes   Cook Time: 10 to 15 minutes   Serves 4

Great appetizer, snack, or extra protein at a low-carb meal.

¼ **cup canned tuna, drained**
2 **ounces cream cheese**
½ **tablespoon heavy cream**
½ **teaspoon lemon zest**
   Salt
   Ground black pepper
8 **large stuffing mushroom caps, clean, towel dried**
2 **tablespoons olive oil (or oil spray)**
   Paprika

Preheat the oven to 350°F.

Combine the tuna, cream cheese, cream , lemon zest, and the salt and black pepper to taste. Using a fork, mix until smooth.

Spoon generous portion of the mixture into each inverted mushroom cap and sprinkle lightly with paprika.

Set the mushroom caps in a shallow, oiled baking pan and place in the oven for 10 to 15 minutes.

Serve warm or cold.

CAESAR IN A PINCH

Prep Time: 5 minutes *Cook Time: 0 minutes*
4 packets (makes 3/4 cup dressing each)

We make this salad dressing in large batches and store it in the freezer until we need it in a pinch. We add olive oil and lemon juice (or vinegar) as indicated below and—voilà!—we've got a great low-carb dressing or dip in seconds.

2 ounces cream cheese
4 teaspoons grated lemon peal (zest)
1 teaspoon oregano
2 teaspoons dried basil
1 teaspoon garlic powder (*not* garlic salt)
12 tablespoons grated, dry packaged Parmesan cheese
½ teaspoon black pepper

Combine all the ingredients in a medium bowl. Mix until well blended.

Divide the mixture into 4 equal servings and put each in a separate foil packet. Place all 4 packets in a ziplock freezer bag.

Store in the freezer for no more than two months.

When you're ready to make Caesar salad dressing in an instant:

Blend or shake well in glass jar:

1 packet Caesar in a Pinch mix
½ cup olive oil
¼ cup lemon juice (or vinegar)
   Optional: add 4 anchovies mashed to paste and blend well again

Makes ¾ cup of Caesar dressing. Store in the refrigerator. Serve chilled.

LOW-CARB ITALIAN FLATBREAD

Prep Time: 6 minutes   Cook Time: 10 to 15 minutes   Serves 4

At one of the hotels in Disneyland Paris they serve the most incredible high-carb flatbread. We consider it an attraction almost equal to Space Mountain. Here's our low-carb equivalent that you don't need a passport to enjoy.

½ **cup green beans, grated**
½ **cup green pepper, minced**
½ **cup celery, minced**
1 **teaspoon salt**
2 **eggs**
1 **cup mozzarella cheese, grated (low-fat or regular)**
3 **tablespoons olive oil**
   Dried basil, oregano, cayenne, and/or paprika to taste

Preheat the over to 375°F.

In a colander, set over a deep plate, toss together the green beans, green pepper, celery, and salt, and allow to drain for 10 minutes.

Run water through the colander to thoroughly rinse the salt from the vegetables; then squeeze well to remove excess moisture.

Combine the vegetables in a bowl with the eggs and mozzarella cheese.

Add basil, oregano, cayenne, and/or paprika as desired.

Coat 1 medium baking sheet with 3 tablespoon olive oil. Press the vegetable mixture evenly onto the sheet, smoothing over the entire area.

Bake until lightly browned and crisp (10 to 15 minutes).

Serve warm or cold, plain or brushed lightly with Pesto Sauce (page 224).

PESTO SAUCE

Prep Time: 4 minutes   Cook Time: 0 minutes   Makes 1¼ cups

We brush this authentic green sauce on the Low-Carb Italian Flatbread (recipe included in this chapter) or toss it with fresh low-carb vegetables.

1 **cup fresh basil leaves**
2 **cloves garlic**
¾ **cup olive oil**
¼ **cup Parmesan cheese, grated**
⅛ **teaspoon salt**
¼ **cup pine nuts or walnuts (optional)***

In a blender or food processor, purée the basil, garlic, and olive oil.
Blend in the cheese, salt, and, if appropriate, nuts.
Use immediately or seal tightly in an airtight jar.
Store in the refrigerator up to a week.

BEDEVILED EGGS

Prep Time: 4 minutes   Cook Time: 0 minutes
Makes 8 stuffed egg halves

We love these as a quick breakfast treat or as a side dish to a low-carb meal that needs something special to perk it up.

1 **teaspoon dried basil**
4 **hard-boiled eggs, cooled, shelled**
¼ **cup chopped cooked chicken or canned, drained tuna**

---

*Optional ingredient. Include only if permitted on your particular low-carb or controlled-carb eating program.

½ **tablespoon ared mustard**
Olive oil (or mayonnaise)*
Black pepper
Paprika
Lettuce or spinach leaves

Cut the eggs lengthwise and remove the yolks. Arrange the egg whites on a cookie sheet or large serving platter.

In a medium bowl, mash the yolks with dried basil. Combine with the chicken or tuna and mustard.

Add the mayonnaise or olive oil as needed until the mixture can be mashed smooth. Add pepper to taste.

Spoon the yolk mixture into the cavities of the egg whites. Sprinkle with paprika.

Serve chilled on a serving tray lined with large lettuce or spinach leaves.

---

*Use mayonnaise only as permitted on your program.

Index